THE HOMOEOPATHIC APPROACH TO AUTISM

ALSO BY PETER TWOHIG

A Vitalistic Approach to Homoeopathic Medicine
Case Management as a Clinical Technology
Introduction to Isopathic Prescribing

THE HOMOEOPATHIC APPROACH TO AUTISM

Peter J Twohig

WARBURTON

Warburton Press
Wyoming NSW Australia

Warburton Press
PO Box 9305
Wyoming NSW 2250 Australia

First Published 2021

ISBN 978 1 922470 06 5 (paperback)
ISBN 978 1 922470 09 6 (ebook)

Cover illustration: Peter Twohig, *Ecce 1*
Visit Wildhomoeopathy.com

For Jason and Tycho

Though we do not wholly believe it yet, the interior life is a real life, and the intangible dreams of people have a tangible effect on the world.

James Baldwin, *Nobody Knows My Name*

Contents

Introduction

Melbourne in 1948 was a very unforgiving world – it was 'sink or swim', so I pretended to swim, and I still am. In common with everyone on the planet, I grew up in the occasional company of autistic people who did not know they were autistic. Some of them were friends, and I myself was one of them. What they had in common was that they tended to avoided the crowd, were often extremely sharp (those who weren't were often relegated, some of them to very sad places indeed) and enjoyed doing strange things. They also had a tendency to exhibit and develop neurological problems, e.g., epilepsy. Often, they were bullied and abused, especially by teachers. Some were dyslexic, some physically awkward, some were hyperactive – the list goes on. But not one of them was recognised as being autistic – that is a recent phenomenon.

By the time I had begun to practise homoeopathy I had met a great many autistic people – hundreds – yet I still did not know how to recognise them. And as long as I was in practice that continued to be the case, though I unknowingly treated many of them, with varying results.

I wrote this book because the homoeopathic literature on the subject is seriously lacking, and what little information there is often flawed and based on misconceptions, despite the efforts of a small number of fine homoeopaths who speak and write on the subject.

There are six main problems with the clinical homoeopathic approach to this neurodiversity as it exists:

- it confuses autism (including its frequent and various presentations) with its common comorbidities[1]
- it implies that there is only one version of autism, when in fact there is *one for each autistic person*
- it lacks special references in the homoeopathic materia medica[2]
- it treats autism as predominantly a childhood phenomenon, when it is really a lifelong experience
- it implies that autism is curable, when that is a category mistake
- it does not (as far as I can tell) address the maintaining or aggravating issues (I do not call them *causes*, despite strident literature to that effect).

The third of these is outside the scope of this book, though I have sought to offer suggestions in Part 4 – *Homoeotherapy*.

Objectives of current book

This book aims to:

- increase the homoeopathic practitioner's awareness of the phenomenon of autism

---

[1] Strictly speaking, autism has no comorbidities, as it not itself a 'morbidity'. However, the species is well-represented in the neurological epidemiology.

[2] These could indicate constitutions.

- offer a general approach to the autistic patient in the clinic
- suggest therapeutic solutions to autistic anxiety (which is ever-present and which has various presentations)
- describe common autistic comorbidities
- suggest therapeutic solutions to common presentations of autistic comorbidities.

Also, I hope the book will go some way to dispelling misconceptions the reader may have concerning autism. I don't expect to do a complete job here for the simple reason that I have entertained all of them at some time despite being myself autistic, and I'm still working on it. Thus, the knowledge grows.

What I can say is that, as autism is an interior way of life it is only describable by the autistic individual himself, whose description will necessarily be unique. Thus, there are approximately 156,920,000 unique descriptions currently available!

The book does not aim to suggest cures for autism, because autism itself is not a clinical disorder (though palliation of stress-related presentations may be in order, as they come with the territory). Neither does it aim to cure comorbidities, though the spectrum of these has not been described, and many of these may be susceptible to the similimum as a palliative.

Also, this book does not seek to fully educate the practitioner on the subject of autism, as this has only recently begun to be discussed openly and with enthusiasm by the autistic community itself (excluding psychologists and psychiatrists, of course, who define it as a brain pathology). Finally, this book is not meant to be in any way inclusive of or a replacement for the fine research and discussion going on all around the world; it is simply a small offering for a large community.

Technological innovations

Occasionally, I make use of a technical and conceptual innovations introduced by me in the *Homoeopathy 2.0* series. When these appear for the first time their sources will referenced in full. Thereafter, I will make use the abbreviations shown in *Abbreviations* (below).

Organisation of the book

Part 1 is an introduction to the nature of autism and an explanation of how it impinges on literally everything the autistic client says, thinks, and does.

Part 2 provides an analysis of the therapeutic matters to be taken into consideration, and therapeutic rationales.

Part 3 provides a discussion on the nature of potency, its influence, and selection, and a suggested approach to posology dosing).

Part 4 suggests homoeopathic solutions to the treatment of the autistic patient:

- preparing a therapeutic strategy
- taking the neurodivergent case, and awareness of issues
- prescribing, patient instruction, and follow-up
- constitutional therapy for autism itself.

Part 5 Provides a limited suggested materia medica for the neurodivergent patient.

The particular suitability of homoeopathy for the treatment of autistic patients.

Homoeopathy assumes that people are much more sensitive to medicine than they think – or could even imagine. Autistic people are invariably much more sensitive to phenomena than *neurotypicals think* – or could possibly imagine. One is led to wonder, therefore, if neurodivergents may be especially sensitive to homoeopathics when compared to the usual patient. In fact, my personal experience is that this is indeed the case, and I will return to this point.

Also, autistics crave relief from the unwanted stimuli, and often those stimuli are internal, that is, sensations indicative of internal processes of the kind that the neurotypical experiences as part and parcel of everyday life. The Homoeopathic Repertory was made for these situations.

Three caveats for the practitioner

First, do not attempt to treat the autistic patient until you have acquainted yourself with the nature of autism. Ignore this advice to the detriment of your patient.

Second, remember at all times that your autistic patient is not a human in the usual sense – at least he may not regard *you* as a member of the same species as himself – and may have experienced a lifetime of insult, abuse and misunderstanding. At the very least he will be traumatised. Forget this for even a moment and he will know.

Finally, remember that your patient (or his parent) may not be aware that he (or both of them) is autistic. It is not your job to break the news to him – unless he has asked for an explanation. Remember that autism is not a medical condition.

Note on Preceding Homoeopathic Books

In 2020 I published Book 1 in the *Homoeopathy 2.0* series: *A Vitalistic Approach to Homoeopathic Medicine* (referenced in the text with the abbreviation VA), which provided:

- a distillation of wisdom in the area of contemporary homoeopathic philosophy along vitalistic principles
- an introduction to a revised homoeopathic technological model along classical lines.

In 2021 I published two further books in the *Homeopathy 2.0* series. The first of these: *Case Management as a Clinical Technology* (referenced in the text with the abbreviation CM), provided:

- a detailed implementation of the principals enunciated in Book 1
- a guide to the vitalistic way of practising classical homoeopathic medicine in the clinic
- a revised homoeopathic technology specially designed to achieve improved results in cases of chronic disease
- case analysis, repertorising and potency & dosage advice, from the first consultation to the final review

- strategies and therapeutic guidelines for the management of notoriously difficult classes of case
- a number of conceptual innovations and revisions.

The second of these: *An Introduction to Isopathic Prescribing* (referenced in the text with the abbreviation IP), provided:

- a theory of group disease (including its displacement of miasmic theory)
- an introduction to the principles of isopathic technology using potentised remedies
- strategies and therapeutic guidelines for the management of detoxification
- possible protocols for the management of prophylaxis
- a set of non-curative protocols for treating certain categories of commonly seen disorders

From time to time, I might reference the above books where I think the allusion could have relevance.

Special features

Chapter outlines

Each chapter is preceded by a list of contents, to assist in previewing the sequence of topics.

Key concepts

Key distinctions, when they appear for the first time, are in italics. They are also defined at the end of the chapter in which they first appear, and in the general glossary at the end of the book.

Further reading lists

These appear at the end the book. These are not reference lists, and their contents may contrast with the author's views, sometimes to the point of disagreement. However, the author will have taken note of them.

Abbreviations

Throughout the text, the following symbols and abbreviations are used:

<	(Causes) aggravation, worse for…
>	(Causes) amelioration, better for…
ADHD	Attention Deficit Hyperactivity Disorder
ASD	Autism Spectrum Disorder
C	Centesimal scale of potency
DSM	Diagnostic and Statistical Manual of Mental Disorders (also DSM-5, the fifth edition)
K	Korsakovian scale of potency
LM	50-millesimal (quinquagintamillesimal) scale of potency
M	Thousand (on the centesimal scale of potency)
X	Decimal scale of potency

Also, many remedy names appear in their commonly abbreviated style, for example, *Sol-t-a* for Solanum Tuberosum Aegrotans.

Dosages

Unless otherwise specified all dosages given in tables and example sets are understood to be ascending collective doses, for example, involving plussing or the like.

Nomenclature

The *sources* of remedies are referred to in their common or, if they have one, their scientific style, for example, silver nitrate, *Arnica montana* (Leopard's Bane), *Tuberculinum bovinum.*

Actual remedies, that is, potentialised medicines, are with a few exceptions referred to by their Latin names using initial capitals, for example, Argentum Nitricum, Arnica Montana, Tuberculinum Bovinum.

Potentialised medicines (also referred to as simplexes) are referred to by their remedy names followed by their potencies, for example, Argentum Nitricum 30C, Arnica Montana 10X, Tuberculinum Bovinum 10M.

Remedies collectively are referred to as the homoeopathic materia medica, whereas the homoeopathic pharmacopoeia (regardless of version) is referred to as the *Homoeopathic Materia Medica*, or simply, the *Materia Medica.*

The Index to the *Homoeopathic Materia Medica* is referred to as the Homoeopathic Repertory or simply the Repertory (regardless of version), and occasionally is uncapitalised, for example, 'his repertory of choice'.

In keeping with common clinical parlance, I refer to recognised comorbidities of autism, despite autism not being itself a medical phenomenon.

In this book I shall occasionally refer to autism, neurodivergence and neurodiversity as if they were interchangeable, though neurodivergence may include other forms of neurodiversity, including putative pathologies.

Male gender pronouns are preferred (except when inappropriate) to preserve textual elegance.

Part 1 The Nature of Autism

1 Autism as a Special Neurodivergence

The Autistic Subspecies

An autistic is a very high-entropy human. Unlike a neurotypical he does not hum along in a steady state, expending energy economically. Instead, he is forced to expend it as best he can, given the unusual configuration of his divergent nervous system. A key characteristic of his is *iteration*.

Thus, on any day, he might seem to be psychotic or manic, or might actually be comatose, desperate, or epileptic. Or he may be completely absorbed in an amazing idea, which may or may never see the light of day, and may or may not make sense to observers, if it does. But it may make sense to him. Often, he will engage in repetitive activities, which will enable relaxation. He will eventually realise that, if he is going to succeed he had better attempt to fit in; often, though, that is an uphill battle: *life* is an uphill battle.

A homoeopathic remedy *also* is a very high-entropic, highly iterative creature. Unlike its mother substance, it is not content to express itself in the laziest way possible. Instead, it wants to make things happen in its unique way. For any given patient it can be relaxant, excitant, or analgesic. Diluting and energising it only make it more determined to show the depth of its genius.

These two unorthodox creations were made for each other.

Autism not a disease or medical condition

Autism is not a disease or medical condition. Thus, it is not a disorder[3] (though it can be disabling) . The fact is that autism is a special form of neurodivergence that is intrinsically benign and not medically problematic.[4]

That said, autistic people typically suffer from having three problems:

- They are commonly treated as if – at their best – they have something intrinsically wrong with them.
- They are hypersensitive to the neurotypical world, that is, its people and its artificialities.
- They are usually anxious, to the point that they do not function well. (That may be said to be the main concern of this book.)

Moreover, autistics typically are plagued with certain neurological problems – most of which have been classified and will be discussed in this book under the heading of comorbidities – for which homoeopathic solutions will be

[3] Autistic Spectrum Disorder (ASD) is the popular misnomer: autism is neither a spectrum nor a disorder. Another is Asperger's Syndrome.

[4] Concerning its inclusion in the Diagnostic and Statistical Manual of Mental Disorders (DSM; latest edition: DSM-5, publ. 2013), a publication of the American Psychiatric Association for the classification of mental disorders, I have no kind words.

discussed. That may be said to be the second concern of this book.

Stressors

On any day the autistic person has to deal with four kinds of stressor:

- social stressors
- environmental stressors
- internal stressors
- the vicissitudes of life,

all of which are unwelcome.

Typically, the level of anxiety of an autistic, even on a good day, is anywhere from high to extremely high, and on a bad one can be literally unbearable, which may prompt an extreme response, for example, an autistic *meltdown* or a *shutdown*. It might also cause a known comorbidity to suddenly rocket to a high level, for example, in the form of a grand mal.

Identification and Occurrence

The emergence of autism

In 2016 US National Centre for Health Statistics reported that the frequency of autism was 1 in 36. This means that everywhere you look you will see autistic people, most of them getting by with no formal identification of their neurodivergent nature. You will have patients, friends, colleagues, and probably family members who are autistic. You went to school with them, studied medicine with them (they make excellent homoeopaths), and possibly were attracted to them and married them (as this is a common autistic experience).

However, until quite recently the distinguishing of an autistic taxonomic group had not been made. Yet, throughout history autistic people have run the risk of being tortured in mental institutions, cruelly put to death, or subjected to 'medical' procedures designed to prevent them from expressing their individual beauty and divinity. That still goes on.

Then, when the distinction began to be formed, it was applied to males. Still later, its occurrence – especially in females – was consistently underestimated. We can now, as I do, not distinguish between males and females. Autism may even be a distinct human species. It is certainly a distinct neurodivergence.

Identification as a social group is helped by thinking of an 'average' autistic, of course, and that is unavoidable. However, there is no standard autistic. The fact is that every autistic is unique, and would not be surprised to hear it, either. To him, the uniformity is on the *outside* of their kind, that is, in the neurotypical population: equally inconsiderate, equally unimaginative, and equally silly, because that view tallies with his own (usually unfortunate) experience.

The emergence of autism as a phenomenon was due to three factors:

- the correct identification of autistic people
- increasing neurotoxicity

- the general rise in compassion.

Neurotoxicity

As for the second factor, neurotoxicity, that is the result of the poisoning of the environment, which is what neurotypicals do best. The effects on neurotypicals are predictable and sad indeed; the effects on neurodivergents are far less predictable, and may be more devastating, because their nervous systems are more sensitive. A homoeopath with an autistic patient needs to be aware that the patient is not only a uniquely neurodivergent human, but one who has been poisoned.

And yes, there will also be a history of trauma – there is always trauma.

Compassion

The realisation that most if not all autistic people have been traumatised in a way or with a frequency that will not let them rest is the result of sheer compassion. We do not like to hear it, but we have the opportunity, for the first time in history, to do something about it, and we are.

The Autistic Spectrum vs the Spectrum of Support

The autistic spectrum

As a matter of nomenclature, or at least usage, note that there is no such thing as the 'autistic spectrum' (which means that there is no such thing as Autistic Spectrum Disorder). However, the idea that there is a spectrum of autism is entirely wrong. The fact is that every autistic is experiencing life in a unique way which is not spectral. Thus, the experience he describes will be special and intimate. It is also essentially invisible, because it is interior in nature.

The autistic support spectrum

There *is* a spectrum of need for support, of course, and your patient will be on it, just as your neurotypical patients will be on it, especially disabled ones. I have made this distinction because so many of the neurodivergents one sees are disabled in some way, especially children. As adults they may find a way to minimise or hide their disability, in which case we may think of them as being not so obviously on the spectrum of need for support. Also, they may be in need of no support at all (though, at the very least it is common to find neurodivergents taking central nervous system drugs).

Autistic Features

Diagnostic features

In order to be thought of as an autistic, one should have the following features:

- Deficiency in social/emotional reciprocity (the give and take of social intercourse)
- A lack of nonverbal communication, including eye contact and gestures
- Difficulty in the area of relationships, including their development, maintenance and understanding of them
- Repetitive behaviour
- Restricted interests.

In addition, the autistic subject would have any two of the following:

- Repetitive speech, body movements or movement of an object

- Insistence on sameness
- An intense special interest
- Hypersensitivities.

When did autism appear?

Autism has probably always been around, though, owing to its small incidence, historically small and isolated populations, and the habit people had of destroying children they did not like the look of, it does not turn up in historical records. However, there have always been places for autistics in seminaries, monasteries and universities.

In recent years, owing to an increase in reporting, the rate of occurrence is rapidly increasing. That is because we are now in an age of virtually universal communication. Even if, as I would assert, there has been a recent aetiological explosion due to toxins, one would expect the occurrence to level out eventually, even if only due to factors intrinsic to the cause itself, for example, a downturn in the reproduction of autistic people, an increase in their morbidity, or a reluctance of parents to be use medications known to compromise the human gut biome and the immune system.

Autism in the sexes

It was long thought that there were many more autistic men than women. However, the numbers are in fact equal. The main reason for the original disparity was found in the phenomenon of *passing*, that is, the habit all autistics, to the extent that they are able, of pretending to be neurotypical in order to avoid social stigma. This is something that women are better at, for the reason that, for a woman not passing can mean social death. Luckily the female world contains a richness of social cues.

As these girls grow up they tend to conduct research into social situations, writing *scripts* that they have seen used by others, and which they will practise. Thus, the social interaction that girls spontaneously enjoy may be followed more or less rigidly, which can give them an appearance of being controlling. To avoid getting things wrong, and because they know that their scripts may lose currency, they flit in out of groups.

This is not a problem with boys, because joining in games does not usually require structured conversation, just an understanding of rules, which is something autistic boys excel at, even if they might not be physically adept.

The typical autistic woman observes and learns (and at the end of the day is sick and exhausted, usually without knowing why). However, even now that the cat is out of the bag, so to speak, you will be hard-pressed to spot a female autistic who is *masking* (to use the parlance), so that I predict that most of your neurodivergent patients – at least those out of early childhood – will be male.

The autistic male, on the other hand, more readily finds his niche, and if it is not a social one he does not care or even notice, more often than not. He has had his fill of bullying and stress, and is content to adopt a low profile, say, behind a computer screen. In his formative years, he does not succeed in blending in, so his parents might compare him unfavourably to his sister, who instinctively knows that she must adopt certain social behaviours if she is to perpetuate the human species.

A girl who is autistic may prefer to play with boys, as she will then experience less pressure to conform and compete. Also, an autistic boy may prefer the company of girls, as they will be less obtuse and unkind to him.

While both girls and boys create imaginary friends, girls are far more elaborate than boys.

Autism in groups, including families

Autistics tend to cluster, which explains the tendency of nerds to congregate (à la The Big Bang Theory). But go to a football match and you will see few of them. That is because they eschew crowds, and because to an autistic teams seem to do everything the hard way, that is, by cooperating, and because crowds don't seem to do anything at all, whereas your average autistic is a very busy person. His idea of relaxation is *doing something*.

Autistic families also tend to contain autistic clusters. It is common for an autistic to come from generations of autistics, and therefore to give rise to more generations. One reason for this is that they tend to attract similar friends, and of course marry them. Similarly, the siblings of autistics may also be neurodivergent.

Diagnosis and misdiagnosis

It is incorrect to think of autism as something to be 'diagnosed', because it not a medical disorder. On the other hand, this is the term that is universally applied to its identification. In this book I shall be using the word 'identified' instead.

Until recently, autism was often confused with bipolar disorder, borderline personality disorder, tantrumism, etc. But owing to the DSM, it has come to be seen as a distinct condition, albeit a medical one. Even so, a moment's thought will show that very few people in the world are aware of their autism (and, therefore, the possible major cause of their unhappiness).

Professional assessment

I do not advocate treating the autistic patient as if he or she is ipso facto ill. The homoeopath will realise that the presence of signs and symptoms discussed in this book will be sufficient to indicate autism, and proceed accordingly. Usually, however, the patient will be a child and will be brought along by a parent who already knows that the child is autistic, nearly always because the child will have been assessed by an expert of some kind.

Life stages

The younger autistic child

For infants the early signs of autism include late development, especially late speech, and lack of face recognition. (However, speech will occur naturally at the appropriate time for the individual child.)

Also:

- The child may not respond to his name, or seem to recognise anyone.

- He may line things up, for example, toys, horizontally or vertically.
- An early indicator of autism is sudden retrogression, especially in speech, usually in response to some kind of intervention, for example, vaccination. It is this common phenomenon that has given rise to the suspicion that vaccines can actually *cause* autism.
- He may never quite get the hang of reading (dyslexia), or may never learn to read at all.
- He may learn to walk quite late, and be extremely clumsy (dyspraxia).
- The autistic child may never make eye contact; for him to do so would be painful.

Late 'diagnosis'

From the medical point of view, a late diagnosis is regarded as one that is not made until the age of four. Plainly, this is ridiculous, when you consider that most of world's autistics have never been identified at all.

The older autistic child

- Speech may not occur until quite late, e.g., the age of twelve.
- He may be particularly awkward.
- The autistic child may never grasp the fundamentals of arithmetic or mathematics (dyscalculia), but may find it necessary to invent his own – *often superior* – systems.
- Social skills may be wanting for the whole of his life. A lot of this may stem from his distaste for touching others or allowing them to touch him.

- Also, the things others take for granted in social events: perfumes, food smells, tobacco smoke, noise, singing, quaint actions and sayings, may be to him disturbing, overwhelming, illogical, unnecessary, foolish, offensive, or all of the foregoing.
- He may become a collector.
- He may make notes about everything, or about his special interest, e.g., car numbers.

The autistic adolescent

Adolescence, especially puberty, will vary from difficult to hellish, and often is accompanied by depression, migraines, or grand mal seizures.

Also:

- He may always be more awkward than his peers.
- He may never get the hang of such things as shaving or she may never cotton on to cosmetic application.

The typical autistic adult

He does not know about autism, and he does not care. Also:

- Often he has *plain face* (a deadpan expression).
- He does not easily look you in the eye. He may therefore seem shifty.
- He is restless.
- He is easily startled.
- You do not warm to him.
- He may present primarily with one of the known comorbidities, e.g., epilepsy.
- Typically, he is photophobic.

- He has very pronounced desires and aversion.
- He is used to craving carbohydrates.
- He may also have a fondness for alcohol or marijuana, to assuage his stress.

Patients who are unknowingly autistic

Most of the autistic patients who are unaware of their autism will go unrecognised by you (unless you are yourself autistic). There's nothing wrong with failing to recognise them. They probably know nothing about autism. Hopefully, the information contained in this book may help you find the similimum for their presentation.

Executive Functioning Difficulties and Cognitive Inflexibility Eye contact

Eye contact is usually painful for autistics, who prefer not to engage in it. Autistics will commonly wear sunglasses which for them serve a dual purpose, most of them being photophobic.

Paradoxically, autistics make great speakers and lecturers, because they regard the faceless mass before them as just that. Similarly, they may enjoy speaking to a camera, because it is not a person, but a machine.

Introversion and extroversion

Some autistics seem to be greatly introverted, and some extroverted, with many alternating. Autistics are prone to having ADD or ADHD, and these greatly add to the autistic picture when present. Also, many autistics are depressed or in pain, e.g., from strong light, a lot of the time. You will probably see autistic patients who are *masking* strongly (unless they are still learning), so you may never see the genuine article.

Meltdowns

A *meltdown* is a loss of emotional control and equanimity, resulting in childlike state resembling panic or tantrum. This is the result of an overload of stress, more common in women, and usually brought on by the stress of passing, or maintaining one's cool.

The homoeopath will probably not witness a meltdown in the clinic, but it definitely puts one in mind of a few well-known manic remedies. Remember, though, that an autistic meltdown is not a manic episode or a tantrum. It is more akin to a seizure in that it will eventually run its course. In any case, it signals the end of the interview.

Memory difficulties

While many autistics have phenomenal memories, especially long term, autistics typically have problems following instructions and retaining short term memories. They also may forget faces (prosopagnosia). They do tend to do well at remembering codified text, e.g., rules. For that reason, they make good lawyers, programmers, etc.

Shutdowns

An emotional *shutdown* will look like a severe depression, though it will pass. I have only witnessed these in males. A male who is shutdown will not communicate – because he may not be able to – and may simply absent himself from the place, if he is able. If your patient shuts down, you will get no further.

Other sensory overload issues

Autistic burnout

Autistics are especially prone to total sensory overload, in all areas, e.g., noise, smells, etc. Usually, they will learn to avoid them. To that end, they will wear noise cancelling headphones, sunglasses, etc. Many of them avoid shopping malls etc. Sensory overload is probably a universal problem for autistics, and is seen in autistic burnout, when the whole experience of daily life becomes overwhelming, requiring a forced withdrawal.

Aversions

Autistics have many aversions, some quite strange, particularly with regard to clothing and food, though nothing may be excluded. This should assist repertorisation. Many of these aversions are related to their heightened senses of taste and smell. All autistics are averse to the mere thought of certain things, for example, textures, shapes, colours, sounds, etc, not to mention inexplicable things, surreal events, etc, which will never come to light, and must remain part of the furniture of their internal world.

Verbal information processing

Many autistics have great difficulty hearing and saying certain words, phrases, voicing concepts, and so on. They may appear to have a sensory problem, while actually having an information processing problem. Verbal processing overloads occur rapidly for such people, and they may appear to be functionally deaf and mute as a result.

Distinctive activities

Stimming

Autistic 'stimming' (from self-stimulating behaviour) is different from neurotypical stimming which comes and goes. Autistic stimming only ceases for brief periods, usually when *passing* (passing as neurotypical) is necessary. It usually takes the form of repetitive movements, e.g., shivering, hand flapping, leg or foot movements, etc. It may involve doing something painful, e.g., tongue biting, and can even lead to self-harm.

Any form of stress relief is covered by stimming. However, having said that, almost all abnormal behaviour by autistics involves stress handling. Stimming has earned autistics a reputation for being weird, if not downright unattractive. Yet it is neurotypicals who have the problem.

Repetitive activities and actions

Autistics typically are adept at repeating actions without becoming bored, and in fact, find it relaxing. When the action is completely meaningless it may qualify as stimming. However, such repetitive types of activity as long distance running may be quite attractive to them. An autistic may find working on an assembly line quite relaxing, and just what he needs to fill in the time.

Special interests

When something captures the interest of the autistic he may give his attention to it as if it was the only thing in the world worth attending to. Often a new object of interest will instantly become his fascination – or *special interest,* to use the common parlance – and may remain so for a short or long time. I have often felt that homoeopathy is such an interest for me, though there have been many others, and I look forward to many more.

It should be noted that a special interest is not a hobby – that is one of the many normalomorphisms wrongly (and often patronisingly) attributed to autistics. It is more of an obsession.

The fact is that autistics have throughout history routinely achieved stratospherically in many fields. Not only do they not think (process thoughts) in the way that neurotypicals do, they may not *understand* the neurotypical way of thinking, which explains why they often struggle at school, despite having intellects superior to and greater appreciation of their subjects than do their teachers.

The possession of special interests is one of the hallmarks of the autistic. It begins in childhood, and never fades. It may be something as simple as collecting Lego pieces, or it may be as complicated as writing computer games.

Other forms of neurodivergence discussed

In Parts 2 and 4 there is discussion of the common comorbidities of autism: ADD, ADHD, gastrointestinal disorders, and other neurodivergences, all of which usually occur independently of autism, but which, when added to it make life very difficult indeed, and throw the autism itself into greater relief.

KEY CONCEPTS

Burnout Complete exhaustion as the result of overwhelm, usually due to the effort of passing, with inability to make decisions.

Masking Changing one's personality to conform to social pressure.

Meltdown Uncontrollable loss of emotional equanimity on the scale of a tantrum.

Neurotypical A neurologically normal human.

Passing Presenting oneself as neurotypical.

Plain face A deadpan expression commonly seen in autistics when not masking.

Shutdown A complete loss of activity, resembling depressive episode.

Special interest Something an autistic takes an interest in to the point of obsession.

Stimming Self-stimulating behaviour, typically leg movements or hand movements used to reduce stress.

2 Autism as a State of Human Life

The Neurotypical View of Autism

The mythos

Autistics are sick and need to be treated

This is the typical held by the fearful person, and yet is the *neuro*typical view. I can't help taking this opportunity to advocate for acceptance here, not acceptance of autistics as a lesser species, but as humans who must function differently to get by in a society not of their making, the keyword being 'must'. Autistics must not, therefore, be treated as if they are intrinsically sick.

As for normality, multiple surveys have shown that autistics who have an opinion on the matter would have no wish to be neurotypical. From the autistic point of view that world looks pretty unexciting. Of course, losing the comorbidities would be tantalising, especially for the epileptics, but just the thought of all the small talk one would have to engage in if one were to become neurotypical is enough to settle the matter, at least for those who can control their seizures.

Autistics are like Rain Man

The film Rain Man was partly based on the life of Kim Peek, a non-autistic savant with FG syndrome, a rare X chromosome-linked genetic syndrome. Notwithstanding, savantism, as it is known, has been reported in about one-third of autistics.

Autistics are easy to spot

Actually, many autistics can pass for neurotypical if they put their minds to it, and they do because neurotypicals often find them intensely inconvenient and embarrassing, and can make their lives misery.

Until autistics learn to pass for neurotypical, which occurs in girls long before boys, they are typically bullied and shunned. The solution adopted by most of these children is to go it alone.

The fact is that it usually difficult to tell whether a person is autistic just from his behaviour unless he betrays himself, which is often the case with children, or unless he is disabled in some way. Thus, mature autistic persons are often aware that they are at risk of self-betrayal, and may go to some pains to prevent being bullied and maintain some degree of social acceptance – a phenomenon known as masking.

Masking is the way autistics 'pass' (for neurotypicals). Masking is universal in autism – of this more later.

Autistics are disabled

While this may be true of many, especially young children who may be unable for example to speak or to read, they are usually able to get by quite well if they get the assistance they occasionally need. The fact is that what works best for autistics is acceptance and assistance, not ablism. All autistics know the pain of being stigmatised – that pain is unnecessary.

Autistics are unintelligent

That is simply not borne out by historical achievements and vocational correlates.

Autistics are insensitive and lack empathy (and are therefore bad)

The main problem autistics have in dealing with neurotypicals and their world is their own enhanced sensitivity and empathy, which borders on the supernatural, but can be maddening. (It can be extremely handy for the autistic homoeopath, of course.)

Autistics are unfortunate

Disability aside, the autistic might take the view that it is the neurotypical who is unfortunate, if unfortunate is taken to mean dull.

Autistics do not understand the way things are supposed to be done
He understands – the question is: does it make sense? As a side note, many autistics have careers in areas of technology (Gr. *tekhnologia*: systematic treatment). An autistic can always think of a better way to do something. Neurotypicals refer to this as 'thinking out of the box'. Autistics just call it thinking.

Autistics are bad, and need to be punished and corrected
Unfortunately, this has been the predominant world view for many centuries and still is. Autistics do not need to fit in: it is society that needs to change.

Autistics are unwilling to be part of society and must be normalised and integrated.
I am sure that there are many autistics who might wish to fit in, if only they knew what that meant, and we know that many fine actors have managed to pull off this feat. However, the autistic way of life it not about fitting in so much as it is about getting by. They are all gifted in some way, even if that way might seem trivial to most, and 'normalising' a genius whose gifts might benefit humanity is definitely not a good idea.

I should add that, as the autistic son of an autistic father, and the father of an autistic son who is himself the father of an autistic son, I have an appreciation of the difficulties faced by parents, siblings, co-workers, friends, teachers and other fellow humans.

The Autistic View

The autistic view of neurotypicality

I have come to think of autistic humans as members of a separate species of human, mainly because I believe that is more in tune with their own view of the human race. To the autistic, the neurotypical human is definitely so strange that he might as well be a member of a different species: he does not seem to truly appreciate his own world, his friends, or even his dog.

He does not realise that he is surrounded by the possibility for fun and games, and is only interested in winning, not as a game but as domination, judgement, and invalidation. The autistic is perfectly willing to validate the wonder of a crack in the footpath, especially if he can classify or draw it. In fact, he may consider cataloguing it in a Book of Footpath-ology.

The autistic in the world of neurotypicals

Where do neurotypicals fit into this picture? They do not. They want autistics to be like them, that is, to stop being autistic, when that is simply a sign of ignorance. They do not realise how fortunate they are to be entrusted with the care and friendship of these sensitive creatures. For autistics are a gift to the world. However, even though neurotypicals can never understand what it feels like to be autistic, they can give their autistic cohabiters the thing they need most: freedom, and where it is required, loving assistance. Freedom and love are two things that the typical neurodivergent may not, historically, have received.

The neurodivergent finds living in the world of neurotypicals unusually difficult. It appears to the autistic that neurotypical life revolves around small talk, truth withholding, lying, cruelty, vanity and pointlessness in general.

It may not occur to him that the popular activities of the neurotypical, e.g., fishing, partying, and the art of seduction, are fun or may serve some deeper purpose, e.g., self-aggrandisement. He may see them as, respectively, frightening fish, participating in torture, and making it difficult to get what one wants. Thus, he may view politicians as criminals, psychiatrists as frauds, and police officers as gangsters. On the other hand, he may be so fascinated by highly regulated tasks and systems that he can think of nothing better than becoming a train driver, an entomologist, or a programmer, at least something he can do alone.

No one is more adaptive than an autistic. He adapts to the incredible craziness of normal human existence – at least to the extent that his neurophysiology permits – by copying others and continually recreating his persona to match, much like a trained actor. Naturally, the autistic child is unable to do this, although the autistic adolescent girl is typically much quicker on the uptake than her male counterpart. Of this more later.

The autistic person does not like what passes for normal human life: he tolerates it – unless, of course, something soothing is in progress, e.g., his cat (when invited), his favourite food (when other, often indefinable, conditions are right), his favourite music (which may be odd and must not be interrupted).

Many of the problems experienced by neurodivergents stem from the fact that the outside world presents certain difficulties for them. It is too noisy, too smelly, too garish, to shiny, too sudden, too mindless and too dangerous. There is too much silliness, not enough logic and not enough word-keeping and punctuality. Nothing seems to have the perfect texture, either visually or tactilely, especially clothing. And everything is hazardous.

The younger autistic child is very trusting indeed, but emerges from early childhood having learned that being hurt once is enough, and becomes self-reliant, even at the cost of non-participation. Thereafter, very few others are considered worthy of trust, perhaps one or two members of the family, but probably no more. To extend that trust further would simply be too difficult a feat to manage, like juggling knives.

Interestingly, the autistic person will probably have at least one autistic parent, and at least one autistic sibling. Also, he may attract at least one autistic friend. He will tend to marry another autistic: better safe than sorry.

His observations of neurotypicals leads him to conclude that they:

- are insensitive
- are bad, cruel and bullying
- aren't too bright
- tend to do everything the hard way
- do not know what fun is

- do not understand the beauty of repetition, pattern, form, mensuration, collection, number, or synthesis.

Of course, this may not be the case.

Being autistic myself, I do not think I like the narrow neurotypical world, with its rules that don't work, its cruelty, its solutions that embody failure, its art that only imitates, its music that often lacks soul and originality, its humour that is purely shallow and insubstantial, its armies that do not appreciate the sheer possibilities of their gorgeousness, their games that are no fun to play.

The autistic's view of his bodymind

The autistic's bodymind does not function properly. In some departments, however, it may seem to work *too* well, for example, in the olfactory department. In other departments it may fail to perform as the neurotypical's does, for example, in speaking or moving smoothly. Others may observe this and comment on it, causing the autistic to spend long hours attempting to improve his 'mask'.

Masking is an activity that all autistics engage in, with varying degrees of success. Many autistics become so good at it that they are able to find work as professional actors, for example, Sir Anthony Hopkins.

Experiential differences

The autistic experiences a richer reality than the neurotypical. His brain senses more, and therefore has more data to process. Left to himself, the autistic will deal with this in the same way that all humans do: by making a space, and working with the data he is interested in, and not with the data he is not interested in. That may be the whole of his process. He may not be interested in working on secondary data later, as neurotypicals often do. He may see this as pointless. He will narrow his interest in order to narrow the data stream, because he is always going to focus more intently.

Neurotypicals see this as obsession and, when it relates to people themselves, rudeness, because of the modern moral myth that everyone – and everyone's every thought – is important. To the autistic that is patently false – if it worth a moment's thought in the first place.

The net result of the data processing experience is that he finds the world of non-human phenomena to be intensely interesting, and immediately – from childhood – makes it his business to appropriate an interesting bit (it can be a large bit – witness Bill Gates) for further play. He knows from childhood that if he attempts to play the human game on the same terms as the neurotypicals, he will not have fun, so he makes sure that he owns the game. That is why so many great achievers have been autistic. Unfortunately, however, the autistic experience of the world has to begin in childhood, as with all humans, and for the autistic childhood can be a nightmare.

Life on Planet Earth

Special difficulties

The autistic is an internal creature. He is usually better at thinking than doing. He is therefore often awkward –

dyspraxic – a failure at getting things done, but a brilliant success at dreaming up patterns. Thus, he is particularly easy to find in the ranks of programmers, mathematicians, physicists, engineers, and scientists. His patterns may not have any practical application, but that does not detract from the fun of creating them. (I had in mind Escher when I wrote that.)

The neurological evidence points to them possessing brains that solve problems faster because they have no choice, having less neurons, at least in the early developmental phase of life.

The autistic person (and patient) may also appear to be uncooperative, diffident, anxious, superior, or otherwise unsociable. This is what causes them to be disliked, and to dislike others. Combine their lack of social skills – they neither possess them, nor particularly wish to – with their natural tendency to regard 'human beings' (as they often think of neurotypicals) with suspicion or distrust (more often than not from years of being treated badly), and you have a patient to whom you have difficulty warming, even if you want to. I have heard autistics say that they often feel that they are on the wrong planet.

The reason why the autistic might come as across as a malcontent, outsider or loner is that this world was not made for one such as him, and he knows it. He is your neighbourhood Vincent Van Gough, if you like.

The autistic (female, especially) may be plagued by suicidal thoughts her whole life. She may be highly intelligent, lonely, stressed (from camouflaging herself), lack social support, and may self-harm.

Neurodivergent children

Then we have the special problems faced by parents of neurodivergent children. The dimensions of their problems are, I venture to say, unimaginable to neurotypicals, and even to their neurotypical parents.

On top of all this – for I do not discount the special difficulties society has with coming to terms with neurodivergents – there are the actual medical challenges – I refer to them as comorbidities, though autism itself is not a morbidity per se – especially epilepsy. It is the homoeopathic treatment of these medical challenges which are the subject of this book.

Finally, there is the special problem of how autistic people who are intellectually handicapped may be identified and assisted. I do not pretend to have a solution.

Autistic characteristics

Socio-clinical characteristics

Attachments

Autistics, especially children, will often attach themselves to a particular object, far beyond what would seem reasonable in a child. Sometimes they keep these attachments for life. You may witness this yourself. An autistic may not be separated from such an object; his equanimity may depend on it.

Empathy

Autistics are natural empathics. They are commonly maddened by their realisation of the pain and emotion of others, and will find it convenient to remove themselves from the source, or to enter a state of distraction, for example, using sound or movement. In the clinic, the autistic patient will empathise with the practitioner as if he could hear his thoughts and have his emotions. All of this will go unnoticed, but it could have a deleterious effect on the consultation. In particular, the patient may be particularly sensitive to danger and threat, because that is what he has become attuned to.

Executive functioning difficulties and cognitive inflexibility

We use our executive functioning skills for getting thing done and multi-tasking. We also use them for switching tasks, resisting impulsiveness and handling day-to-day challenges. This is also related to memory difficulties and emotional control problems. For an autistic, change will not only present challenge, but can be literally unbearable.

Fears and phobias

Fear is the dominant emotion in the life of the autistic. He is afraid of everything, sometimes of his reflection in the mirror, or his shadow. He may be afraid to answer the phone or open his mail. He may even be afraid of television. He is especially afraid of the unexpected. The 'Fears' rubrics in the repertory will all be relevant at some time or other. He will always be found to be afraid of something odd, often something which could not possibly be guessed.

Introversion

Most autistics are introverts, though this not the rule, and often they swing between introversion and introversion, with shyness being extremely common. On the other hand, an extroverted autistic who has worked out the secrets of masking can be hard to spot. What will usually give him away is his talkativeness. All the loquacious remedies are relevant.

Memory difficulties

Autistics often have phenomenal memories, bordering on the supernatural, though sometimes they have specific amnesias, e.g., prosopagnosia (face-blindness). They may also have short-term memory problems leading to executive functioning difficulties.

Verbal information processing

Neurotypicals do not talk only to provide information: they also do it to socialise. Socialising can be quite painful for autistics – frankly, they do not see the point – and the irritating nature of its content can be quite confusing, because their brains take everything to be literally true (when it has been my experience that practically none of it is). This does not mean that autistics do not understand humour. They do, but first they have to parse it, an unconscious process, to be sure, but still one that requires an additional time and energy-consuming step. But once an autistic cottons on to the humour game he may play it with genius. My favourite example is Jerry Seinfeld.

Distinctive Activities

The following activities may be stress relief strategies, or they may simply be special interests.

Counting

Autistics often compulsively count, sometimes out loud, sometimes in odd arithmetic arrangements, e.g series. Sometimes they make notes of their tallies.

Journaling and note-making

Autistics often keep notebooks, sometimes on a variety of subjects, and sometimes from an early age. Journaling helps them make sense of the otherwise drab and meaningless world. They may also draw in their journals, or paste tickets, receipts, etc. Often the autistic will maintain notes of his special interest, e.g., of observations. For example, he might be a price-watcher or car-watcher, collect cars numbers, collect the frequency of certain words he hears, and so on. He might also create rules and write them down. He likes rules.

Organising

He may organise constantly, to the extent that his home or room is a model of organisation. If he has bookshelves, their contents will be arranged. His whole life might be arranged, if that is possible. To the autistic, there is nothing worse than losing control of the world. He may also organise the people around him, which can make him extremely unpopular. Remember that all of his behavioural characteristics are based on fear.

Passing

Autistic people usually do a fair amount of passing, that is, passing for normal. It's a stressful business, and can be both rewarding and unrewarding. For girls and women, it is essential to successful socialising. The downside is that the pent-up stress can be literally unbearable and require extensive downtime or relief, often in the form of a meltdown. This is a strategy that children cannot adopt, with the result that their apparent tantrums often can be continual. When is an autistic passing? Whenever he is near other people.

Pattern making

The autistic loves patterns, and will spot them and impose them freely. He is often able to solve patterns, anagrams, cryptograms, etc, with blinding speed. Many movies are based on their ability to do this. A Beautiful Mind is one such movie. Another is The Accountant. Autistics see patterns everywhere, and take their ability for granted, rarely if ever realising that very few people can do this. Imagine going into a Persian rug shop and not being able to distinguish any patterns. How drab it all would seem. Now imagine going into a field of ordinary grass and being mesmerised by the patterns. For an autistic nothing is random. Many of the greatest mathematicians were and are autistics.

Poetry and fiction writing

The autistic loves stories, because he may be possessed of the ability to hyperfantasise, a feature of some visual cortexes, and because he can imagine much better versions of the world than the perceived one. You need to bear in mind that the autistic patient finds the world as it is highly unsatisfactory.

Problem solving

Above all, the autistic is a problem solver. For neurological reasons, he has been forced to solve problems with fewer neurons from infancy. He has a natural ability to visualise novel and ingenious solutions to problems. Before becoming a naturopath and homoeopath, I worked for many years as a management consultant, systems analyst and database designer.

Programming

Many autistic adults are programmers. They like computers, and computers like them. Many of them are online gamers.

World and character creation

May autistics live in a fantasy world which they often spend years constructing. Some of these people end up writing book series based on their fantasies. Autistic children routinely invent best friends for themselves. It's a wonderful solution.

Part 2 Therapeutic Considerations

3 Therapeutic Complications

Introduction

There are two types of therapeutic complication in the autistic presentation: typical autistic comorbidities and the general group of what may be thought of as obstacles to cure, or more correctly, obstacles to therapeutic success.

I have come to regard autism itself in two lights: the light of anxiety, which is present in every autistic and varies only in intensity, but never in chronicity, and the light of comorbidity, whose appearance is so frequent as to be expected (though that is not, I think, the rule).

In this book, I shall address the comorbidity itself, e.g., ADHD, only when it is co-present with autism, and not when it is the sole presentation. There are actually a great many neurodivergent comorbidities, many of which are either not covered in this book at all or at least not covered in depth. I have never heard of a comorbidity being completed eliminated by any form of autistic therapy, so I will assume that palliation is the best that may be hoped for using homoeopathy.

The class of obstacles to therapy is headed by gastrointestinal disorders, which are legion. Gastrointestinal disorders will only be mentioned in passing in the book, and I will give them some attention in an Appendix, however I will not devote homoeopathic coverage to it, as it is a vast subject in its own right. The practitioner is therefore advised to apply the similimum as he sees fit, or to palliate.

Having said that, he may also wish to apply the principles of *isopathy* to its treatment if he suspects that detoxification is required (which in my experience it always is). The subject of isopathy will be covered in a later chapter.

I will not treat the anxiety state that invariably appears in autism as a comorbidity, but as the main presentation, and will cover it separately in Part 4.

Frequent Comorbidities

The aim of this book is not to discuss the common autistic comorbidities, but to list them with the minimum distinction, to facilitate later parts. I should begin by saying that is quite common for autistic patients to present with a complex of comorbidities, none of which might seem to have a distinct aetiology.

The leading comorbidities are:

Attention Deficit Disorder (ADD)

This is characterised by:

impulsiveness
disorganisation
problem-solving difficulties
time management difficulties
difficulty focusing on tasks and multitasking difficulties
restlessness
planning difficulties
being easily frustrated
being easily distracted
inattentiveness.

Attention Deficit/Hyperactivity Disorder (ADHD)

The key symptoms are decreased attention and hyperactivity. Other symptoms include:

aggression
excitability
fidgeting
irritability
lack of self-restraint
persistent repetition of words or actions (though several of these are common indicators of autism itself).

Cognitive symptoms
Absent-mindedness
Difficulty focusing
Forgetfulness
Problems paying attention
Short attention span

Mood symptoms
Anger
Anxiety
Boredom
Excitement
Mood swings
Depression
Learning disability.

Gastrointestinal disorders

Gastrointestinal problems are experienced by almost all autistics, especially children, and there is a direct correlation between the severity of an autistic presentation and the severity of gastrointestinal issues (from dysbiosis). Such concomitants as headache, noise sensitivity, and irritability, are all usually related to constipation, diarrhoea and abdominal pain.

The manifestations of leaky gut syndrome may include:

Autoimmune disease (Systemic Lupus Erythematosus (SLE), celiac disease, Crohn's disease, rheumatoid arthritis, multiple sclerosis, psoriatic arthritis, vitiligo, osteoarthritis)
Brain and cognitive issues (from blood-brain barrier malfunction), e.g., brain fog, headaches, memory loss, frontal lobe inhibition (leading to depression, anxiety, attention deficit)
Chronic fatigue (often associated with fibromyalgia, poor nutrition, inflammation, decreased brain function and immune system issues)
Cravings, especially for carbohydrates (from dysbiosis)
Digestive problems (diarrhoea, constipation, bloating, irritable bowel syndrome)
Immune system disorders
Multiple allergies (and food intolerances)
Nutritional deficiencies
Skin rashes (acne, eczema).

Leaky gut syndrome must be addressed at the very start of homoeopathic treatment. If dietary steps are to be taken, they must run alongside homoeotherapy.

Other common disorders

Aggression

Alexithymia – difficulty identifying one's own emotions or those of others

Anxiety (more common in girls)

Depression (more common in girls)

Dyscalculia – difficult understanding and manipulating numbers

Dyslexia – difficulty reading

Dyspraxia – difficulty planning and coordinating movements

Epilepsy (present in approximately 39% of autistics – more common in girls)

Immune system disorders

Irritability

Neurodevelopmental problems

OCD (more common in girls)

Paranoia

Post-traumatic Stress Disorder (PTSD)

Prosopagnosia – Difficulty recognising familiar faces

Sleep disturbance

Speech delay or difficulties

Note that many of the comorbidities listed above, while being accepted as distinct by mainstream medicine, are probably signs of leaky gut syndrome, and are therefore susceptible to cure or at least amelioration by adopting dietary measures.

Acute, Chronic, and Pseudochronic Disorders

The concept of group disease

In the *Homoeopathy 2.0* series I introduced the concept of *group disease* as a way of explaining the aetiology of disorders which were not endogenous. Thus, a group disease is a disease of a group, whose members share it via specific vectors. It corresponds by a factor of scale to an individual disease. The concept displaces the miasm theory.

Thus, for example, vaccinosis is treated as a group disease, as are the communicable diseases, and all pseudochronic diseases (see below).

The elimination of group disease from the individual is achieved by the administration of the vector in potency, a protocol known as isopathy. This procedure has the effect of weakening the energistic bond, that is, morphic resonance, between the individual and the enrolling *morphic field*.[5] The result will be a degree of palliation with a diminution of symptoms as therapy continues. The group disease concept will be used as appropriate throughout the book.

---

[5] In an attempt to construct a theory which unifies epidemiology, materia medica, and pharmacodynamics, further explained in Twohig, P 2020, *A Vitalistic Approach to Homoeopathic Medicine*, Warburton Press, Wyoming NSW. I have adopted Sheldrake's hypothesis of formative causation, which explains how species may learn and evolve through the interaction of morphic fields, by morphic resonance (Sheldrake, R 1985), *A new science of life: The hypothesis of formative causation*, 2nd ed, Anthony Blond, London).

Is autism a group disease?

The question is put because matters of remedy scalarity could have a special impact on therapy for autistics, and because group disease is not curable with homoeotherapy (and neither is autism). But the answer is no: autism is not a group disease, unless we regard group disease as having a genetic axis as well as a social axis (and I do, but I think that a different kind of vitalistic therapy, e.g., of a constitutional nature, might be necessary to address that – see chapter 12).

Simply, a group disease is always defined by its specific vector, which is theoretically removable. In fact, this was the basis for miasmic therapy.

Acute disorders

Vaccinosis

The main acute disorder to look for in autistics is probably vaccinosis, that is, an illness that follows the receipt of a vaccine or so-called vaccine, a condition to which autistics are particularly susceptible, owing to their natural hypersensitivity, especially to toxins. Indeed, I have treated children who were reportedly symptom-free prior to being vaccinated, when they seemed to suddenly become autistic.

I regard these patients as having been already autistic, and having been exacerbated, despite the evidence of their parent, simply because autism is a condition that a person is born with.

Nevertheless, remedies in potency can work wonders for these patients. The *Materia Medica* provides remedies, both homoeopathic and isopathic.

Immune reactions

These are common, often due to a bowel dysbiosis-related compromised immune system.

Childhood diseases

Autistic children tend to over-react to the usual childhood infections. However, they are usually easier to diagnose as a result.

A communicable disease is an example of what I have come to think of as a *group disease* (classical: *miasm*), not an individual disease.

Intervening disorders

These acute disorders crop up with more than usual regularity with autistics, especially children, for a number of reasons arising out of the autism itself. They may result from:

epidemic and childhood diseases
food intolerances
injuries
lack of sleep
seizures.

It may be necessary to discontinue current homeopathic treatment in order to attend to them (to avoid multiple prescribing). However, note that if the current therapy is isopathic, concurrent medication may be carried out simultaneously. The protocol will be addressed in the chapters dealing with potency selection and posology.

Chronic disease

The paediatric patient may present with chronic disease, and if that is the case he will need to have that condition distinguished from his presenting disorder, if it is different. In children, the chronic disease may well be neurological in nature, in which case it may be thought of as an autistic comorbidity. Otherwise, you can treat that condition, or not, depending on the parent's request.

It is not uncommon for chronic diseases to be associated with autoimmune disease, in which case they should always be treated as primary, and not secondary, as such a disorder will affect the whole case from start to finish. It might even be possible to dispel the condition, if detoxification is successful.

Since the mid-1990s there has been an epidemic of autoimmune disease, especially:

Alzheimer's disease
asthma
celiac disease
Crohn's disease
multiple sclerosis
thyroid disease
Type 1 diabetes.

Also, there have been first world epidemics in:

ADD/ADHD (1 in 10, most on medication)
allergy (1 in 4)
asthma (1 in 10)
autism (1 in 36)
cancer (1 in 2)

dementia (1 in 1)
depression (1 in 2)
diabetes (1 in 4)
obesity (1 in 3)

largely as the result of the destruction of bacteria in crop soil, destruction which results in damage to the gut lining, the blood brain barrier, and every other organ that is protected by intercellular tight junctions.

Naturally, these disorders are also occurring in epidemic proportions in neurotypical patients as well, with the result that many (especially children) may be difficult to distinguish from autistics in their mentals.

Miasmic therapy

Prescribing a miasmic nosode for a chronic disease is not recommended. First, such a miasmic is not a homoeopathic but an isopathic, and therefore will cause detoxification at a level that might not be predictable or necessary. I have found gratuitous nosode therapy to be harmful to the integrity of the case, as these can waste time and may cause an unwanted proving.

Naturally, any nosode which has been proven will have recorded symptomatology, and thus may be pre-checked. You will find that its prescription is unwarranted. The only possible exception would be where the miasmic may be confidently prescribed as a homoeopathic (i.e., as the similimum).

None of the foregoing applies to the acute miasmics, of course, which may be prescribed to eliminate the aftermath of a childhood disease, a situation that more often occurs in adults.

Aetiology

You will find that it unsafe to prescribe on aetiological grounds, as autism (and its neurological comorbidities) are usually genetic in origin. If, however, you suspect some other aetiology, e.g., chemical, then you may prescribe isopathically. The neurodivergent adolescent or adult who takes recreational drugs (except cannabis, of course) will have obvious contributory aetiology.

Constitutional therapy

The prescription of the patient's constitutional remedy is, as far as I can tell from reported cases and online sources, routinely used as a substitute for the similimum. That practice is to be eschewed except where the similimum actually turns out to the constitutional remedy, otherwise it will result in a disordered case (see below). The fact is that throughout one's life, one may be prescribed the similimum with the desired effect without ever requiring constitutional therapy.

Having said that, I must go on to say that there is a place in homoeotherapy for the constitutional remedy, and that will be discussed in Part 4.

Pseudochronic disease

Aetiology

Pseudochronic disease is neither self-resolving (acute disease) or permanent (chronic disease) but is typically continual in the presence of its maintaining element, which may be thought of as a toxic substance (though not necessarily a physical one, e.g., noise).

All autistic people have experienced pseudochronic disease, and for children, who do not have control over their own lives, this can be the source of unbearable stress.

The autistic adult, on the other hand, is usually able to do what works. Of course, knowing that one is autistic and understanding the ramifications of that is a tremendous advantage. However, most autistic adults will never gain that knowledge.

Solution

Unless permanent damage has occurred, pseudochronic disease may be cured simply by removing the maintaining cause. Unfortunately for the autistic that is not something that society would deem desirable.

Society does not want the autistic to experience his unusual life free from interference: it wants to intervene, often in the name of submissiveness, if not conformity. It wants the neurodivergent to cease his stimming, put on a happy face, and knuckle under. Your mission, should you choose to accept it, is to help your autistic patient be a happy neurodivergent, not an unhappy neurotypical.

The secret to dealing with pseudochronic disease is to identify the cause of the patient's toxicity and remove it. In the case of the neurodivergent it is usually a dietary problem, invariably carbohydrate. But it may also be a whole swathe of food additives.[6] The treatment of pseudochronic disease is something that will not wait.

Further Complications

Multiple aetiologies – the complicated case

A complicated case is one having several aetiologies, which is often the case with adults, but is less frequently so with children. Naturally, if your patient is autistic and does know it (or whose parent does not know it), this will certainly be an aetiology. Do you say what you suspect? I would not advise it, unless it is a natural question to bring up in the circumstances. The fact is, a mother may not want to hear that her child is autistic (and anyway, you may be mistaken). An adult, on the other hand, may be greatly relieved to have that knowledge.

But quite apart from the contributory role that autism always plays in pathology, there is the question of what else could have caused the patient's problem. There is bowel dysbiosis, of course – that is a given. And, of course, there is the presence of some other contributory factor, e.g., allopathic medication. All the aetiologies must be gathered together and analysed as, for the autistic none of them can be discounted. Basically, if he mentioned it, it is relevant. Case analysis will be discussed in Part 4.

---

[6] If you are not up to assessing the patient's dietary intake, you must refer him to a naturopath.

Faulty prescribing – the disordered case

A disordered case in one in which incorrect homoeopathic prescribing has occurred *without correct antidoting*. This will usually if not always be the case when a patient is referred by another homoeopath who has tried and failed to make headway.

The only path forward is to antidote in reverse. It will be necessary to take the case afresh, and carefully prescribe the similimum. At some time during therapy you will get back on the right track simply by means of sound prescribing.

Iatrogenic disorders

The autistic patient has usually received some form of treatment from non-naturalistic practitioners, perhaps from allopaths, or worse, from aversion therapists. He may have received electric shocks, drugs designed to modify his behaviour, various forms of restraint, injections of vaccines and other substances. He may be so traumatised that he is reluctant to share himself with the practitioner. That is good, as you will now have a solid starting point, especially if you know the probable reason.

Iatrogenic disorders invariably require some kind of detoxification, if only that which naturally result from the similimum being given.

Further complicating factors

The homoeopath himself

A major complicating factor in the treatment of the autistic is the belief system of the homoeopath. The homoeopath must interpret the case at hand and incorporate it into his own belief matrix, without prejudging. That's a big enough ask for the routine case, but the neurodivergent is a special kind of human, eminently vulnerable and yet exquisitely powerful.

He is capable of achievements that are meaningless to the neurotypical. Whatever he does he does in a unique way, outside the defined field, and less inaccessible to others, including his peers. What cannot be appreciated is the special way in which he makes sense of the world. It may be nonsensical to the alien observer, yet it is for the single inhabitant of that world intensely interesting. However, he does not want to – perhaps can't – explain himself.

History of abuse and post-traumatic stress disorder

If the patient has attended school he has been bullied and beaten (or worse), perhaps by adults (especially if he attended a boarding school, or was 'taught' by Catholic teachers). Thus, there will be scars of one sort or another.

Depending on the events of his life, there will be some degree of Post-traumatic Stress Disorder (PTSD) present, which may have to dealt with or at least taken into consideration. This will definitely be the case if the patient has been in a combat situation in the Army.

This is the fragile yet strange being whose suffering you now behold and who has reluctantly decided to trust you.

The clinical approach to complications

The general approach to complicating factors will be dealt with in the next chapter, but you will see that although these factors may seem to be endless and insurmountable they are not, and may be dealt with by simultaneous detoxification and prescribing to the acute situation.

Do not expect a new and underlying chronic disease picture to emerge, as chronic disease will be apparent early, especially in an older patient. And remember that the autism itself it not a disease picture, but a special human picture.

KEY CONCEPTS

Constitutional, -al remedy A remedy that is reminiscent of the constitution of a patient.

Group disease A disease of a group. It corresponds by a factor of scale to an individual disease.

Isopathy Treatment of group disease by administering a potentised group disease vector.

Isopathic Of a medicine, being made from the same species that caused the disease.

Isopathic prescribing The prescribing of a homoeopathic medicine on the principle that a specific and not generic (that is, similar) match will result in the annihilation of a form of resistance that is identifiable with a group disease. Isopathics are often prescribed for the elimination of group disease

Morphic field Resonant field. See **morphogenetic field**.

Morphic resonance Harmonic attunement resulting in reverberative propagation, and synchronisation.

Morphogenetic field A self-organising and self-remembering, spatio-temporal, vibratory, pattern-imposing, probabilistic field shared by co-resonating members.

Pseudo-chronic disease A category of disease that resembles chronic disease but always is sustained by repeated exposures to a morbific agent.

4 Therapeutic Rationale

Introduction

You cannot, as a practitioner, simply take the whole patient as you find him, and assume that the similimum (much less the constitutional remedy) will do all the work, as he has a complex of problems, most of which are not facets of autism as we commonly define it, but are comorbidities requiring separate interventions.

As we saw in the last chapter, regardless of the prima facie diagnosis, an aetiological analysis will invariably reveal a complex of:

- autism itself (including some irritating factors)
- at least one comorbidity
- at least one pseudochronic disease
- at least one iatrogenic disorder.

Thus, I venture to say that you will not encounter a more complicated picture. The patient may be incurable, but is eminently palliatable. We do not achieve this by 'treating the layers' – that is simply not possible, that being an erroneous concept. Instead, we remove whatever it causing the distress we see and treat the anxiety itself, because that is always present. Then we address the pseudochronic factors.

Other factors to be addressed include:

detoxification
dietary control
lifestyle support
allopathic support.

Luckily, all of these measures may be taken simultaneously – indeed they must.

Homoeopathic treatment of anxiety

Treatment of natural autistic anxiety takes the form of palliative homoeopathy (the similimum) together with isopathy (for detoxification) and constitutional support (as an ongoing measure). In this regard I do not regard identifying the constitution as being an issue, as it is usually a simple matter to arrive at a group of candidate remedies. I'll discuss this further in a later chapter

Removing irritants

Naturally, the first step in treatment is to remove any irritants. With an autistic there can be a huge number of them, and the parent will know them. They must be removed, if progress is to be made. It is no good tormenting the child, then expecting him, perhaps in response to threats or enticements, to correct his behaviour. His behaviour was already correct; it was simply unacceptable to somebody else.

The secret of success is to realise that the environment – and the patient's body's response to it – are unbearable to him. He is hypersensitive to what is outside his skin, and suffering because of something that is going on *inside* it (usually a substance hypersensitivity or a chemical response to a leaky gut). Remember also that his neurotransmitters and hormones are never going to be normal.

Detoxification

The autistic child will invariably be in need of detoxification. All the irritants he ingests (most of which may never be specifically known) are driving him crazy. Their effects are not intermittent: they are ever-present. He will live with them his whole life. No wonder he becomes difficult to live with.

There are two ways to detoxify him: give him a correct diet, and give him homoeopathic (including isopathic) support. Other methods, in which the body is in some way coerced, e.g., chelation therapy, will not improve the situation and will therefore cause harm.

And of course, detoxification must always be accompanied by the cessation of *unnecessary* allopathic drugs.

Homoeopathic treatment of comorbidities

Acute disorders, which is how most comorbidities manifest, must be treated as and when they occur, according to the urgency, and this may have to be a permanent approach to a given patient. Note that the neurodivergent child will often present with intervening disorder, e.g., epidemic diseases, and these will take precedence, not necessarily because they always do, but because of the additional anxiety they cause. In this respect it could be that in any case you will find that prescribing a stress-related remedy will work better than a traditional childhood disease remedy (which might make a better second prescription).

Comorbidities are also exacerbated by toxic load, and to that extent are pseudochronic as long as the exposure is in progress. That is why dietary control is required.

Dietary control

Autistics invariably require dietary monitory, if only because their bodies tend to be deficient in certain chemicals, e.g., neurotransmitters. Luckily, the patient himself will always indicate by his food preferences that something is wrong with his diet (not that his preference for carbohydrates is a positive thing – it is not, as his bowel biome, in its mysterious tribal way, readily attests). The parent of a child with leaky gut syndrome should treat all processed carbohydrate as poison.

This is the main treatment area for autistics, without which attempts at homoeopathic palliation will be useless, and which we will return to in a later chapter.

Dietary supplementation will be required, possibly permanently. I will return to this point.

Lifestyle support

Lifestyle support may assist an autistic, but only if his teachers (if he is a child) understand. If he is an adult he will have already figured out what works and what does not for his happiness to be improved. More often than not, it is refraining – not engaging – that does the trick.

Allopathic support

Allopathic support will be required for some comorbidities, especially epilepsy, for which homoeopathy may not have any effect at all, as the acid test is chemical withdrawal, *which I do not recommend*. Other comorbidities, e.g., ADHD, may respond to gradual chemical replacement with homoeopathics.

Other forms of allopathic support, e.g., acupuncture and botanical medicine are, in my experience, always beneficial to some extent.

Part 3 Vitalistic Pharmacology

5 The Nature of Potency
6 Potency Dynamics
7 Approach to Potency Selection
8 Approach to Posology

5 The Nature of Potency

Introduction

It is necessary to return to basics it we are to treat the autistic patient, because the case will of necessity be complex. We must now therefore revisit:

- the nature of homoeopathic potencies
- the dynamics of homoeopathic medicines
- guidelines for potency selection.

The Nature of Potency

Homoeopathic and isopathic medicines

The nominal potency of a remedy is an indicator of that remedy's power to assist the vital force to overcome its stall and continue to express the central disturbance in a timely manner.

It is important to bear in mind that a remedy exerts its *own* intrinsic curative force. Thus, the *actual medical power* of a homoeopathic as prescribed is always a product of its *intrinsic curative power* and its assigned potency.

Note that, in relation to the individual patient the above formula does not apply to potencies when applied in their isopathic (eliminative) *mode,* whose purpose is not to bring about cure but to eliminate *group diseases* (classical: *miasms*) and their attendant vectors and toxic by-products. An example of this use would be the treatment of vaccinosis with MMR in potency.

In both uses the assigned potency is also a reflection of the vital force on display. Potency should therefore be increased with the dramaticity of the presentation.

The homoeopathic-isopathic distinction is relevant to much of the discussion in this book, and will be referred to from time to time, as necessary.

'Physical' potencies

The curative power of any given 'substance' may be amplified by potentisation, whether that method be shamanic chanting, or succussion and deconcentration. The chemical dilution of a medicinal substance for reasons of safety thus has nothing to do with vitalistic healing per se and would simply be a matter of common sense. Also, to speak of a potency as being physical is a nonsense. Vitalistic medicines are inherently mysterious, as is their use.

Dimensions of potency

The clinical dimensions of (a given case of) disease are:

- *scale*: level of illness, e.g., particular, general, mental, group
- *phase*: life stage e.g., children, adolescents, adults, the dying
- *frequency*: level of vital force apparent
- *velocity*: chronicity.

These may be thought of requiring the following potency solutions, respectively:

- scale of attenuation (potency scale)
- succussions (or equivalent energising ritual)
- deconcentrations (number of dilutions)
- dosage (exposures).

When faced with the prospect of potency selection for the autistic patient two problems arise: how to minimise aggravation and how to match the patient's vital force, and both must be addressed simultaneously. Whatever solution we come up with is made difficult by the way homoeopathics are produced and packaged (that is, with the number of succussions and dilutions locked into scales), making constant prescribing compromises necessary. I am fully aware of the limitations this situation imposes; however, the solution is quite simply to apply the *Golden Rule of Prescribing*:

Match the medicine to the vital force

Scales of potency

Scalarity in vitalistic pharmacy is inescapable. Homoeopaths have found that scalar attenuation can be combined with serial deconcentrations and dynamisations to elicit from remedies their magical medical powers. So which scale is best? The question is moot, due to the way homoeopathics are manufactured. For autistic patients, I recommend the most attenuated scale available, that is, the 50-millesimal (LM) scale, whose base dilution is 1:50, 000. I advocate that scale due to their exquisite sensitivity of autistics, even to attenuated potencies.

Plussing

The only freedoms are afforded to those who serially dilute and succuss – that is, plus – their remedies manually, and instruct their patients to do the same when dosing (using the Korsakovian method). Those practitioners may control the scale. If *plussing* is done properly, that is, rigorously and *consciously*, the results can be astonishing. I emphasise consciousness because it is just that feature of every facet of homoeopathic life that brings the desired-for results.

Non-standard scales

In relation to autistic patients, you may consider that the scales as provided are inadequate, and that you can improve on them – that is the Hahnemannian way, after all. Whatever works will be fine. The only caution I would offer about non-standard scales is that they must be intelligible and reproducible to any homoeopath who later takes over that patient and the case record.

We will return to guidelines for potency selection and matters of posology later in this chapter.

Scalarity of groups

Once again it is necessary to consider scale attenuation in the case of the autistic patient, but for a slightly more different reason. If we use isopathy, we known exactly what kind of toxins will be eliminated – that is the whole point of the therapy – and the sudden appearance of those toxins can be stressful for the eliminative systems, and of course for the mind. For a neurotypical patient this might not be a problem, so we might use a more heroic scale of potency.

However, for the autistic patient the scalarity needed to achieve this effect should, given the heightened sensitivity of such a patient, be more attenuated. Also, the scale of any simultaneous homoeopathic should different.

Bear in mind that all of this vitalistic activity will be taking place against a background of measures designed to restore of bowel health, because these alone could have a drastic eliminative effect.

Potency number (deconcentrations)

As a rule of thumb and consistent with all aspects of vitalistic medicine, the medicine's power should match the patient's vital force. We do not seek to oppose anything about the patient, including his illness or his pathophysiology. Thus, we should use potencies of *low frequency* (potency numbers) in cases of low vitality, and high potencies in high vitality. That is the main consideration in potency selection. Too low, and the requisite *healing gradient* will not be achieved, too high and unnecessary aggravation will occur.

Succussion and life stage

Succussions are directly related to the patient's life phase. Normally, in their selection, we would closely consider:

- aetiology, e.g., a definite vaccine reaction
- relationship of illness to life phase, e.g., measles in childhood
- likelihood of cure.

In cases of autism there might be no hope of cure, however there is extremely high expectation of palliation. Even better, the presenting patient is almost always a child, so we know that, because of the *phase shift* effect shown by all homoeopathics (as palliation proceeds it retrogresses the pathology) the case might not take long, depending on the age of the child, to reach a satisfactory conclusion.

Palliation will have the effect of assuaging acute symptoms. Naturally, it will be necessary to remove the exogenous source of any other problems, if that is possible. In adults that might mean broaching the subject of substance addiction, always a tough ask. In children it will mean discussing allergens, etc. (though children have their addictions too).

Scale-phase compromise

The packaging of standard Hahnemannian potencies entails the linking of succussions, and to some extent, potency numbers (number of dilutions) to potency scales. However, this is not an obstacle to good prescribing. It simply means that prioritising must be done. Thus, the order of importance for child cases is: scale, succussions, potency number – all of which points to the LM scale in a low number.

Chronicity and potency

Dramaticity

The key predictor of cure is always the dramaticity of the presentation. Dramaticity is the outer feature of the bodymind's attempt to overcome its blockage of the vital force. However, in cases of chronic disease, where acute episodes often lack that feature as a differentiating characteristic, cure is not well indicated. The bodymind's rhythmic attempts to create healing crises may weaken over time in intensity, though they may go on forever if left untreated. However, they may not weaken in frequency of their appearance, resulting in the chronic picture.

Dosage and retrogression

We may consider *chronicity* as the nosological indicator of the *velocity* dimension of illness. Chronicity is defined as the time elapsed since the symptoms *first* appeared, that is, regardless of reoccurrences. The pharmaceutical solution to chronicity is *dosage*, where a *dose* is defined as the number of consecutive exposures of the medicine needed to cause the *most recent* episode to disappear. What will follow will be a retrogression to a past acute episode, which will in turn respond to a further dose of the medicine, and so on.

Naturally, each dose will be at a higher potency, as the vital force will be gradually improved.

KEY CONCEPTS

Actual medical power The product of a remedy's intrinsic curative power and its nominal numerical potency.

Chronicity 1. The time elapsed since the onset of symptoms. **2. C of symptoms**. A result of the failure of the life force to complete its timely expression through the organism.

Dosage The amount of exposure to a medicine.

Dose A single exposure or collection of exposures to a given potentialised medicine.

Healing gradient **1.** The natural inclination of the organism to heal. **2.** The inclination to heal that is installed when a potentialised medicine is administered.

Modes of medicinal response There are eight: amplificational, curative, eliminative, palliative, probative, restorative, supportive, and susceptive. (See each, separately.)

Plussing The practice of succussing a medicine before it is dispensed, usually by succussing the medicine bottle 5-10 times, for the purpose of raising its vital force.

6 Potency Dynamics

Homoeopathic pharmacodynamics

The modal dynamics of homoeopathic remedies were outlined in *A Vitalistic Approach to Homoeopathy* (2020). Briefly, homoeopathics may be thought of expressing seven medical *modes of action*: susceptive, amplificational, palliative, curative, eliminative (isopathic), supportive, and restorative, in which they may be prescribed. As this book is not a treatise on homoeopathic philosophy or theory, I will not go into greater detail than is necessary. However, as I will be using some of these terms – they have become a part of my internal homoeopathic parlance – I will take a moment to explain.

Modes may be thought of as the way in which remedies behave as a function of the method by which their intrinsic medical qualities are elicited from them. It has been my observation that a given remedy will tend to have its expression in a particular mode or modes, sometimes in a cyclic way. For example, Plumbum Metallicum tends to have a distinct expression in the *eliminative mode*. While Chamomilla will tend to express its nature beautifully in the in the *palliative mode*.

For the sake of completeness, I should add that I have also identified a non-therapeutic mode, the *probative mode*, which is displayed during a remedy's proving.

Susceptive mode

Initial susceptibility

The *susceptive mode* is that in which the initial effect of the remedy occurs. Occasionally, the healing gradient is immediately achieved, though usually repeated exposures are needed.

Enhanced susceptibility

A patient who does not respond to a single exposure of the similimum will respond to – that is, have his susceptibility increased by – repeated exposures. The practitioner will then have installed the requisite healing gradient, and nothing more will need to be done as long as the curative effect is proceeding.

Persistent susceptibility

A patient who has received the similimum will continue to be susceptible to the same remedy for some time, often until he returns, when he may only require a lesser potency. Incidentally, this is why many practitioners administer the constitutional remedy at the end of a case.

Naturally, there are dependent factors:

- a sufficiently high vital force in the patient
- the *actual medical power* of the remedy
- the *force* of the medicine administered, i.e., the remedy-in-potency
- any supervening toxicity (including allopathic medicine).

Note that prophylaxis is nothing more than the installation of persistent susceptibility in anticipation of a specific illness.

Amplificational mode

The next modal response of the remedy will be in the *amplificational mode*. If the remedy was well indicated, this may be the immediate result of the very first exposure, that is, if susceptibility was achieved instantaneously, otherwise it may require repeated exposures to the remedy. It is always indicated by a visible increase in the symptom picture (which points to the next remedy). It is while the remedy is acting in this mode that homoeopathic aggravation occurs.

The constitutional in amplificational mode

If the remedy given was the patient's constitutional remedy, then the symptom amplification will be the result of an expansion of the vital force generally. In some cases, for example, where the patient's comorbidity is ADHD, this may be alarming. Thus, with an autistic patient the wisdom of leading with the constitutional remedy (unless it is also the similimum for the comorbidity) may be questioned. In any case, caution should be exercised.

It should be understood that in any given case the constitutional remedy and the similimum might not be same thing. A given disease is an affliction of an individual bodymind, and the remedy that neutralises such a disease is the similimum, which acts homoeopathically.

However, a disease that infects a social or human *group* (classical: *miasm*) cannot be removed from the individual by a homoeopathic, though palliation of the visible component of the *group disease* (classical: *miasm*) may be possible, leaving the underlying chronic disease intact, if temporarily ameliorated. Thus, the only solution to such a disorder is the isopathic one.

Isopathy is the 'homoeopathic' solution to all forms of chronic disease, as it neutralises the link between the individual and the group. The visible effect of the isopathic at work is elimination. See *Eliminative mode* (below).

Palliative mode

Fractional palliation

A remedy which was well-selected, though not the exact similimum, will tend to bring about some form of amelioration, which is to the better, of course. However, except when the remedy was the *exact* similimum that amelioration will not be the result of cure, but of *fractional palliation.*

This response is often seen during constitutional therapy and homoeotherapy designed to have a narrow effect, for example, as an *antidote* or for the purpose of first-aid. Palliation is often so successful (because relief from major distress is so dramatic to see) that it can be mistaken for cure.

While there is nothing wrong, per se, with aiming only at fractional palliations in a given case, the repeated use of this procedure using different remedies will nearly always result in a disordered case, as described in chapter 3. In such a case, serial antidoting is usually required.

Emergency use

Notwithstanding the foregoing, in a case where an immediate partial solution is required, for example, in a child who experiences frequent autistic meltdowns, a proven palliative may be required so frequently that the parent has to keep it on hand.

The palliative mode is the main mode of prescribing used for both autistic stress and the leading symptoms of all of the autistic comorbidities, remembering that most of these are invariably the result of aggravations caused by toxins, especially dietary toxins.

Curative mode

Cure is indicated by a return to a state of lasting well-being as far as underlying limitations permit. During the healing process elimination will occur and, frequently, aggravation. These responses will be in line with:

- the closeness of the remedy to the symptom picture
- the potency of the medicine
- the health of the vital force generally.

They will be mitigated by:

- unresolved toxicity
- unresolved bowel dysbiosis
- suppressive medication
- the patient's neurological base-state, which is intrinsic and permanent.

Sad to say, there are medically sanctioned procedures, including electroshock therapy, electroconvulsive therapy, aversion therapy and torture, which are designed either alter the neurological base state or to retrain autistics to act 'normally'. I have witnessed the aftermath of these procedures in patients. Needless to say, they are bound to fail and some cause incurable trauma.

Partial cure

Where there are multiple aetiologies, as are often seen in older patients, the similimum may not match all of the leading symptoms. Its administration may reveal a fresh symptom picture showing some of the original symptoms together with new symptoms. It is possible that, despite continued well-indicated prescribing, complete cure may never be achieved in otherwise curable cases.

The good news is that, as therapy proceeds and the vital force improves, the patient (and the patient's family) will become more stable and happier.

Eliminative mode

Toxic elimination in some form invariably occurs following the administration of any energistic medicine, and is usually accompanied by increased mental and emotional activity (which are also forms of elimination). Although we normally associate the elimination of toxins with exogenous substances (isopathy) it also relates to endogenous toxicity (homoeopathy).

Organic elimination

The organs of elimination that are activated tend to be related to the remedy selected. For example:

Berberis – kidneys
Nux Vomica – liver
Petroleum – skin.

As the internal organs improve in function we observe the elimination of pathophysiological by-products and environmental toxins.

Psychological elimination

There will also be a release of pathopsychological by-products, for example, unwanted habits, ideas and emotions.

The latter kind of release could pose a problem for the autistic patient, and may have to be closely monitored. That is because his whole approach to sensation is to minimise it and to insulate himself from it. Whereas the neurotypical has built-in tolerances that he is always aware of, even if he doesn't like them, the neurodivergent does not.

Neurological elimination

Finally, autistics are in the habit of eliminating stress continuously, for example, by stimming, speaking, and making noises. Thus, even when the patient is about as well as he is going to get, he will continue to eliminate stress in whatever ways work for him for the rest of his life. Attempts to curtail these phenomena will distress the patient.

Isopathic response

Note that the elimination of the presence of a specific group disease (classical: *miasm*), for example, a given vaccine disease vector, is always the main aim of isotherapy. Thus, we can speak of the general aim of the isotherapeutic programme as the elimination of social vectors. That is why the practice of isopathy is relatively straightforward: the correct remedy is always indicated by the source toxin itself, which only needs to be identified and potentised.

Prophylaxis for autistics

The prophylactic preparation of a hypersensitive patient, such as an autistic, is not recommended, for a number of reasons:

- the elimination response may be stronger and may result in include unwanted distress
- it may not be possible to monitor the response

- the correct antidote may not be known, or be at hand.

Notwithstanding that, an autistic who is confident may wish to take a specific prophylactic if, for example, he is about to travel abroad. Naturally, he would also take a suitable homoeopathic for symptomatic palliation, if needed.

Supportive mode

Concurrent supportive prescribing

Because stressed organs of elimination might fail to perform satisfactorily even under the influence of the similimum (and in the presence of autism *all* organs will be stressed), it may be considered necessary to prescribe a concurrent remedy for the express purpose of supporting an organ or system while the leading homoeopathic is running. Such a remedy is called a *supportive, protective, or stimulant* (and will, invariably, be an organ specific in its own right).

For example, Berberis might be prescribed as a 'hepatoprotective' during detoxification, or Thuja might be prescribed as an immune-supportive detoxification during the treatment of *vaccinosis*. (The practitioner will tend to develop a group of go-to supportives as he goes along.)

A supportive remedy should be given:

- in low potency
- at any time with the main remedy
- as long as it is not itself a possible similimum (or it might act as an antidote)
- whenever a suspected toxin is to be eliminated by an isopathic.

Unproven remedies

If the chosen supportive remedy is an unproven sarcode, e.g., Cerebrum, its potency should be kept low, as the effect will be slightly unpredictable from the homoeopathic point of view (though the target organ can be expected to experience an amplification of its efficiency). In any case, the potencies of the two remedies should be widely different in order to separate the energy fields to be addressed.

Herb-based remedies

A special note for highly sensitive patients, especially children: medicines that are based on edible plants, for example, Calendula, will be found to be quite gentle in low potencies, and are therefore recommended highly for autistics.

Restorative mode

In the *restorative mode* cure is typically followed by an unexpected and *new* level of wellbeing. Thus, this may be thought of a level that transcends cure and may be spectacular to witness.

There are three preconditions:

- cure (of the fresh condition) has been achieved
- known obstacles to health are being managed
- chronic underlying disease, for example, osteoarthritis, is minimally influential.

I have described this dynamic mode for completeness: I would not expect to see this level of amelioration in an autistic patient, simply because autism itself is not a pathology. Any claim by an autistic patient (or his patient) that his autism has been cured will be the result of a confusion of the primary autism with its nosological overtones, which can be extremely wearing.

Note

In the treatment of autistic patients several of these modes are of necessity greatly attenuated, especially in paediatric cases, where the patient will often refrain from giving descriptive feedback – at least of a kind that makes sense – and the effect of a remedy may have to be guessed at.

KEY CONCEPTS

Amplificational mode A mode of medicinal action in which the patient exhibits an increase in vitality (resulting in aggravation, if symptomatology exists), often seen after the constitutional is administered.

Curative mode A mode of medicinal action in which the similimum acts.

Eliminative mode A mode of medicinal action in which the patient exhibits increased mental and emotional activity, with physiological elimination. The primary mode of isopathy.

Palliative mode A mode of medicinal action designed to bring about rapid relief.

Prophylaxis Homoeopathic prescribing in anticipation of a disturbance of the vital force.

Restorative mode **A** **m**ode of medicinal action following homoeotherapy in which the patient's post-curative life changes for the better.

Support remedy In a detoxification combination, the remedy prescribed in the lower potency, usually for the support and protection of organs of elimination.

Supportive mode A mode of medicinal action in which the role of the medicine is the support of an organ or system, especially during detoxification.

Susceptive mode A mode of medicinal action in which remedy acceptability, both immediate and persisting, is enhanced or instilled.

Vaccinosis The generic group disease caused by vaccination.

7 Approach to Potency Selection

Guidelines for Potency Selection

Prescribing scenarios

There are, broadly, two prescribing scenarios for potentised remedies: homoeopathic and isopathic. The first of these utilises the similimum to palliate the symptoms of autistic anxiety and comorbidities. The second addresses the symptoms of toxicity, both endogenous and exogenous, and infectious disease (classical: *miasm*).

The underlying assumptions are: that autism and its comorbidities are amenable to palliation, and that autistic patients invariably carry a toxic load that is eminently reducible with the assistance of potentised remedies used as isopathics.

These treatment scenarios are distinctly different, and will be treated as such.

The necessity of concurrent prescribing

The problem that many practitioner have when it comes to isopathy is that they do not realise that it may be deployed simultaneously with the similimum. Also, they may not know how to use isopathy (see below), so they do not, which results in the patient exiting therapy with a toxic overload, underlying chronic disease, and predispositions to certain group diseases (classical: *miasms*). In this book, both protocols – homoeopathic and isopathic – as they may be applied to autistic presentations, are given.

In the face of uncertainty, say, when an inexperienced practitioner does not realise that he is looking at a complicated case, he may prescribe what he erroneously believes to be the similimum (or perhaps, the constitutional remedy, in the belief that they must be the same thing). The result is that the near-similimum might bring about palliation of his autistic patient, which is quite a feat when you think about it, and may be all that could possibly be expected by the parent of the physician.

However, remember that we are dealing with a case of underlying pseudochronic disease, usually with a complex of aetiologies. Inevitably, therefore, they will continue to cause the same problems.

Prescribing nosodes

While an autistic presentation may occasionally attract a proven nosode as the similimum or the constitutional remedy, an unproven nosode should not be prescribed for an autistic presentation, say, as a supporting remedy unless it is done with the intention of eliminating a disease vector, as autistics are hypersensitives.

Moreover, if the physician had decided that the remedy was MMR, or Vaccininum, or a popular nosode, then he has not found the similimum at all, but has prescribed an isopathic, which may or may not cause elimination, which may in turn cause additional symptoms unless accompanied by *supportive* remedies.

Furthermore, if he has decided to prescribe a nosode, for example, Carcinosinum, simply because his Repertory gives it as a remedy for autism, that is not good enough. Quite simply, the case must be taken.

The guiding rule is always to ask: *How might the vital force respond to this remedy?*

Concurrent medication

The practitioner who is not sure what to prescribe as a similimum might be tempted to prescribe two or more remedies at once, possibly as a complex. This is a bad idea, as it will instantly muddy the waters, making it difficult, if not impossible, to unravel the mess.

However, there is a place for concurrent prescribing, and that is either:

- when one of the remedies is designed to act as a homoeopathic (palliative), for example, Pulsatilla, while the other is designed to act as an isopathic (detoxifier), for example, Nux Vomica, secondary, or
- when one is meant be an isopathic eliminative, for example, Candida Albicans, while the other acts as a homoeopathic hepatoprotective, e.g., Lycopodium.

Naturally, the selected potencies in both cases would be separated by orders of magnitude.

Homoeopathic Prescribing

Following are the main situations in which the autistic patient will require homoeopathic palliation. Recommended remedies will be given in Part 5.

Aetiology and the similimum

As I have already said, it is far more difficult to achieve satisfactory results with homoeopathic treatment than it is with isopathic treatment for simple reason that homoeopathy only works if the similimum is identified.

If there is aetiology, so much the better. Homoeopathic prescribing for an aetiology will take place when the patient's parent (as is usually the case) leads with a known cause. In this case the Repertory will suffice. The reported cause will usually be connected to the patient's hypersensitivity.

Note that, if the patient's hypersensitivity is related to food, it will probably have been exacerbated by the presence of toxins, especially due to bowel dysbiosis.

As for potency, it should be kept very low – I recommend starting with 1LM – and, plussed until the healing gradient has been installed.

Anxiety disorders

Every autistic suffers from anxiety, though he doesn't have to. If he is left alone, he will settle into his own low-anxiety state, providing he is allowed to stim freely, is not forced to conform, is provided with the things he needs to keep busy, and is protected from environmental disturbances and irritations. If he presents in the clinic he will be anxious, a condition for which there is an abundance of remedies.

As for potencies, the remedy in potency should match the dramaticity of the vital force. Thus, the rule that I usually advocate for hypersensitives of leading with 1LM goes by the wayside when there is great distress.

Childbirth

The autistic mother-to-be may be extremely well-prepared, because that is her nature. (I have heard of a case where the patient made her pregnancy her special interest.) Also, she will be afraid, not only of what might go wrong, but of being surrounded by medical people. Her experience of 'experts', especially medical ones, might be bad. If she is patronised during her confinement she will be extremely reactive, and could experience a meltdown. There is a simple solution, and that is to cooperate with her. Potencies should, as always during labour, match the dramaticity of the presentation.

Chronic disease

If there is a chronic disease, which is quite often the case with autistic adults, the practitioner should seek to eliminate it in the usual retrogressive steps using the similimum for the acute episodes. The potency will not be problematic unless the patient has an issue with aggravation, when you may never come to an understanding. The fact is that is that, no matter how inconvenient it is, homoeopathic aggravation, even if unintended, is a sure sign that the necessary healing gradient has been installed.

Naturally, isopathy can also be used to eliminate underlying cause, for example, substance sensitivity.

Clinical therapeutics

This is straightforward, and the solution may be readily found. Autistic people have more accidents than neurotypicals, due to dyspraxia and failures of proprioception. Also, their minds may wander (this may be related to seizure disorder). They are reportedly more likely to get food poisoning due to a sensory failure caused by the presence of toxins (due in turn to gut dysbiosis), especially in the mouth and nose, limiting the usual warning sensations.

Constitution

The special use of the constitutional remedy will be discussed in a separate chapter, as it has multiple uses.

Emergency treatment and first aid

Apart from being accident-prone, autistic children are often myopic. In adults one sees an earlier onset of arthritic conditions and immune disorders. The family should have its own first aid kit. The kit should be supplemented over time, as more acute situations arise. I recommend low potency LM remedies, except for acute mentals.

Epidemic (homoeopathic) prescribing

In an epidemic, the autistic child will typically be highly susceptible. When he has frank symptoms homoeopathics will do. For dealing with the underlying disease vector, elimination (classical: *miasmic*) therapy will be needed, and that is best handled by a practitioner. Low potencies will usually do.

Ordeal

Autistics cope well with ordeals they have prepared for. An autistic adult can be stoic and deliberate. However, if something unexpected occurs he may attempt to stick to his plan no matter what, a course that usually leads to suffering. (The autistic does not understand why others (neurotypicals) sometimes break the rules of the game – the beauty of flexibility may escape him.)

However, if the autistic has not prepared or is unsure of what to expect he will suffer in a way that a neurotypical would not understand. The autistic bodymind will attempt to distribute the stress, and fail. The worst outcome will be a meltdown, a shutdown, a seizure, or something similar.

If the nature of the ordeal is clear, then the patient may be able to take the correct palliative with him to take as required. In these situations, the potency should be commensurate with the patient's anxiety level.

Paediatrics

The range of homoeopathics available for the autistic child is narrower than the range for adults because they have not yet fully expressed their bodyminds and because they have not accumulated a long history of medical problems. The usual range of children's remedies is therefore applicable, plus a few that you wouldn't immediately associate with a child. An autistic may respond to his childhood remedies for the rest of his life.

Remember that several of the common contents of vaccines, for example, Aluminium, have been potentised, and may give rise to symptoms – not as indicators of the similimum but because the child has been poisoned.

The usual paediatric remedies are prescribed in low potencies. for example, low LM.

Palliation

Palliation will have the effect of assuaging acute symptoms. Naturally, it will be necessary to remove the exogenous source of any other problems, if that is possible. (In adults that might mean broaching the subject of substance addiction, always a tough ask. In children it will mean discussing allergens, and food issues.)

Phobia therapy

The Repertory will indicate the remedy to be used not only for a particular phobia but for all phobias experienced by the patient – no need to give different remedies. The autistic patient is afraid of just about everything, so you don't have to look far for a remedy. Unfortunately, these remedies will allay anxiety, but that is all: the object will still inspire fear. The author has gone to extreme lengths to neutralise his own myriad fears, and none have worked.

Psychiatry

Whereas the adult neurodivergent has learned that it is best not to share his mentalisings, lest they be mistaken for pathology, the child has not. Couple this with the tendency of neurotypicals to regard neurodivergents as sick (hence the DSM), and you have an emerging picture of prejudice, stigma, punishment and 'treatment', which is something the child should never witness, let alone be subjected to.

It is not surprising, therefore, that many autistic children grow up scarred, frightened and confused, with many eventually experiencing depression. Luckily, the Repertory abounds with remedies for that, though I have not homed in on them for my short materia medica (chapter 13), as there are too many.

Note that potencies should match the dramaticity of the symptoms (*not* the severity). Thus, a child who feels a meltdown coming on (as he grows older the signs will appear) may take a higher potency of a remedy with similar symptoms, while a child who feels a shutdown approaching will attract a completely different remedy, one that may work well with a lower potency.

Isopathic prescribing

The following headings are the main situations in which the autistic patient will require elimination of either a disease vector or a maintaining cause.

Aetiology

Unlike homoeotherapy, isopathy is *totally* dependent on aetiology. In that sense is not essentially a first response to symptoms, but a response to a known cause. Thus, it is possible – even desirable – to use homoeopathy and isopathy at the same time to address, respectively, the symptoms of disease and its pathology. The former application will result in the neutralisation of the vitalistic blockage within the patient, while the second will result in the weakening of the bond of the patient with the causal influence.

If the patient is also being treated with the similimum its potency will of necessity be matched to the vital force. The only caution therefore is that the potency of any concurrent isopathic be placed on a different level, so that if it causes a proving you will be able to see it clearly for what it is.

Chronic disease

A chronic disease is one that will not resolve itself, usually because of a weak or distorted vital force. The patient who presents with chronic disease is usually an adult, and the acutes will be dealt with using the similimum. Children with chronic disease are less common, and will respond to the similimum more dramatically. (Far more common in autistic children is *pseudo*chronic disease – see below).

Note that the usual autistic comorbidities, for example, non-acquired epilepsy, are not examples of chronic disease, though they are easily triggered by influences which should be removed or minimised.

Detoxification

Every autistic patient requires detoxification. They will invariably have been overloaded with:

- allopathic drugs (especially but not only for comorbidities)
- toxins acquired through leaky gut syndrome
- dietary toxins from sugar, carbohydrates and processed foods
- toxins contained in vaccines
- alcohol or recreational drugs (including cigarettes), if they are adults
- allergens, e.g., casein
- unfriendly microorganisms.

A reduction in any of the above will result in an *immediate* improvement. That is said in the full awareness that certain situations, for example, allopathic drugs and substance dependency, may not be amenable to change, or may be intractable.

As for potency, the practitioner should select one that, together with the remedy selected, will begin a specific elimination process. Usually, a single dose of a high potency will be required to start the process.

As there will always be a slight toxic load while healing is proceeding, it will be necessary to prescribe a complementary concurrent remedy, as appropriate. Often that remedy will be a response to fresh symptoms, for example, itching, and will therefore be a homoeopathic. If such a remedy is used it will not interfere with the action of the primary (isopathic) remedy, which will continue to run in the background.

If there is a complex of aetiologies, which is usually the case, then a series of isopathics, each with its appropriate homoeopathic concurrent, may be prescribed, provided, of course that each of the homoeopathics is allowed to complete its action before a different one is given. As with all isopathic therapy, potencies should match the vital force.

Epidemic

An autistic who presents with an epidemic disease having a well established vector, for example, measles, should be regarded as suffering from acute group disease (see below).

Euthenics

Women may benefit from a course of remedies designed to eliminate the effects of past disease, for example, rubella. This is a therapeutic path that may appeal to autistic women, as they tend to have autistic children. The potencies should be given in series in case there is an eliminative effect, and the potencies kept low. Note that the remedies given do not have to be nosodes, though usually they are.

Group disease (Classical: miasm)

The paradigmatic example of the acute group disease is epidemic disease, to which children are particularly susceptible. Such a patient is easily treated using a higher potency nosode together with lower potency supportive remedy. In this case the supportive remedy can be a homoeopathic prescribed on the basis of leading symptoms, that is, a similimum.

In other words, we are not using the supportive to support an organ of elimination, but to support the whole patient (because he will be miserable). The Repertory abounds with suggestions: the appropriate nosode, for example, Morbillinum, is always self-evident.

An example would bc a disease that responds to allopathic suppression, only to return, perhaps with periodicity, for example, shingles. Note that chronicity requires constant dosage adjustment, if one is to minimise aggravation while maintaining the retrogressive effect.

Pseudochronic disease

The leading cause of pseudochronic disease in autistics is poor nutrition, which can result in malnutrition or gut dysbiosis. Most pseudochronic diseases are the result of something being ingested on a regular basis. They all respond to the removal or rebalancing of the offending influence.

Often, supportive homoeopathy is required at the same time, to assuage the symptoms of a temporary spike in toxicity or cravings. Autistic children, especially, react badly to the removal of a food or substance they like, and their response may attract a higher potency support remedy, as a result.

SUMMARY

In each of the above cases the options as they might be applied in an autistic presentation call for particular mindfulness and finesse. The practitioner should bear in mind at all times that:

- the parent may also benefit from the remedy if she is autistic as well
- the potentised remedy may be delivered in any form that the parent thinks will be accepted, including in food and drink (and sweets, if that is what it takes – I always preferred hundreds and thousands)
- homoeopathic potencies should begin as low as possible and always be plussed before each exposure
- in isopathy supportive potencies should begin low whereas eliminative potencies should be considerably higher, to separate the two.

8 Approach to Posology

Introduction

The subject of posology is dosage. It is often neglected or incorrectly applied during the prescription stage, because it is not understood. But quite simply, it has to do with the degree of the patient's exposure to the medicine. If it is not understood during prescribing the patient will tend to unnecessarily aggravate if it is overdone, or fail to experience the intended impact of the remedy in potency if it insufficient. Such failures in anticipation are due to lack of appreciation of the behaviour of the vital force when it is disturbed. Consider the following two dicta of homoeopathy: the dosage theorems.

Dosage Theorems

The minimality theorem

The first dictum has been referred to in classical parlance as the law of the minimum dose. It is not in fact a law – there are no laws in vitalistic medicine – but a vitalistic theorem, which may be restated (in order to make sense) as follows:

> *A disturbance of the life force will be annihilated by precisely the quantum of medicine that will cause the life force to resume its timely expression of the disturbance.*

We may think of the theorem as a rule of *sufficiency*. That purpose of minimum potency practice is to prescribe precisely the amount of medicine required to install the healing gradient, no more and no less. The vital force will then follow its natural inclination to self-heal. The installation is achieved by *dosage*, which governs the way in which the patient is exposed to the remedy at that given potency.

The posoequivalence theorem

The next question is: How may sufficiency be achieved? The answer is: By prescribing a single dose, comprising the number of exposures necessary for the healing gradient to be installed. In other words, we will treat each singular disturbance of the life force with a single dose of a single remedy. Thus:

> *A singular disturbance of the life force will call for a single dose of the medicine that will initiate cure.*

Once the installation of the healing gradient has been achieved, it will need fractional boosting to match the steadily improving vital force, and this is achieved by *plussing* the medicine. Thus, after the initial stage, the remedy will not need to be repeated at the exact prescribed potency.

Note

1. A full discussion of dosage theory may be found in the three books comprising the *Homoeopathy 2.0* series, in particular Book 1: *A Vitalistic Approach to Homoeopathic Medicine*.
2. While these theorems (and others) have been derived from observation of the similimum's action, none may be derived from observations of the isopathic potency, which is not designed to cure.
3. The single dose is always understood to be a *collective* dose, comprising the series of exposures necessary to achieve the installation of the healing gradient.

Dosage Dynamics

Induction of susceptibility

Initial susceptibility

As explained in chapter 6, the first exposure to the remedy in potency always causes the introductory or initial susceptibility. If that did not happen, the remedy would never work.

Enhanced susceptibility

Susceptibility to the remedy will be increased with each successive exposure, resulting in the installation of the healing gradient (if this was not achieved with the initial exposure). That event will be signalled by a slight aggravation, which is due to the remedy beginning to act in the amplificational mode (see below). During the period of escalation, the patient will have been experiencing *enhanced susceptibility*, which will increase with each exposure to the remedy.

Note also that susceptibility is not a function of correctness of remedy selection. This effect may be achieved with any remedy.

Enduring susceptibility

Enduring susceptibility is usually experienced when the remedy has done its work. The patient will then be more susceptible to that remedy in the future, especially if he receives occasional maintenance doses. (The only time we see this mechanism fail is when there is a fundamental failure of the vital force, such as that often seen in the elderly.)

Installation of the healing gradient

The installation of the healing gradient is achieved by dosage, especially in the form of repeated exposures. It is maintained by additional exposures, usually in the form of fractionally ascending potencies of the same remedy, achieved by plussing.

The true power of the remedy in potency is the power to neutralise a blockage of the vital force, in much the same way that a password unlocks a computer. But note that the password does not cure the computer of its inertia: the password has nothing to *do* with the computer, yet when the computer is given a dose of it, its full power may be observed.

Maintenance of the healing gradient

In a sense, we constantly monitor the healing gradient to ensure that amelioration is always taking place. If amelioration ceases, then the patient is either cured or at least partially so, or the isopathic, if we had given one, has completed or partially completed its eliminative task. In any case, the healing gradient may need to be reinstalled.

Results of the inappropriate healing gradient

Scenario 1: An aggravation of the similimum

The patient has, as instructed, taken the remedy until a slight aggravation was noticed. He was given an extra exposure to ensure a positive result. He then displayed an unbearable aggravation.

His courses of action are to either:

- wait for the aggravation to pass, knowing that it will be followed by considerable amelioration or

- take the appropriate antidote (which is unknown until the practitioner sees the symptoms for himself).

Scenario 2: A proving of the isopathic

The patient has taken a remedy designed to eliminate a known toxin from his body. Not unnaturally, he displays the symptoms of a proving of the toxin.

He must be treated with the similimum while waiting for the toxicity to pass.

Scenario 3: A homoeopathic proving

The patient has been given the incorrect similimum, and is displaying the symptoms of an aggravation together with new symptoms that are characteristic of the remedy but not the patient.

He must be given the appropriate antidote to his new total symptom picture before the case can proceed.

Dosage and chronicity

Chronicity – the temporal dimension of disease – is resolved by dosage. Multiple exposures of the medicine will cause acute recent episodes of chronic disease to be palliated, eventually resulting in retrogradual healing. As the vital force improves, it will be necessary to increase the potency used but usually not the remedy.

Repetitive dosing as a solution

It is understandable that a practitioner may wish to avoid prescribing in a potency that will cause undue aggravation, especially in an autistic child. For that reason, he may select an inappropriately low potency. However, that will invariably lead to overly frequent dosing, which may lead to not all of the target symptoms being addressed, or to constant small aggravations which never lead to clear amelioration. The solution is to select a higher potency, one that matches the patient's vital force.

The Dosing Protocol

Posology and autism

Once the healing gradient has been installed it is imperative that dosing be suspended, otherwise unnecessary aggravation may occur. For autistics, especially children, an aggravation can result in a meltdown or an accidental exacerbation of a comorbidity.

Induction of enhanced susceptibility

Naturally, susceptibility to a given remedy will be proportional to the sensitivity of the patient, and this is always a factor with autistic patients. However, as stress always heightens this effect – and the autistic patient will be stressed by the clinical experience if by nothing else – the point and intensity of aggravation may be difficult to predict. Thus, caution is advised.

It should be noted in this regard that a remedy which is high in *intrinsic curative power*, for example, Phosphorus, will always tend to require less exposures of a lower potency before aggravation occurs, while remedies which do not have this characteristic, for example, Lycopodium, will require the opposite. Thus, a forceful remedy, for example, Stramonium, might achieve the desired effect after one exposure, while one of much less apparent action, e.g Baryta Carbonica might require a series of exposures before a healing gradient is installed. Note that, in both cases initial susceptibility would have been achieved immediately.

How to maintain the healing gradient

Plussing

If the effect of the remedy has worn off, then exposures may be resumed, providing the medicine has been plussed, that is, succussed. Thus, all subsequent exposures of a given remedy are given in increasing fractional potencies which together are known as the collective dose. Remedies may be plussed simply by shaking them vigorously. Note that the number of succussions does not change the potency number, for example, 6 LM, only the vital force of the medicine.

Divided dose

If we wish to attenuate the scale of the medicine we might place a drop of the medicine in a glass of water, then succuss it again, perhaps by vortexing (vigorously stirring). This is a common way of dosing a hypersensitive person.

Extended divided dose

Further scale and potencies can be achieved by repeating the process, by pouring out the contents of the glass, then immediately refilling it, and vortexing it, giving a Korsakovian potency. This could be done with every successive exposure.

Split dose

If the remedy is prescribed before and after a particular event, for example, sleep, then the dose is called a *split dose*. Often, this is done to avoid an event which might interfere with the remedy, e.g aggravation. However, just as often it is done to avoid antidoting a concurrent remedy.

Continued dosing post-treatment

This may be done in two circumstances:

1. If the remedy worked unexpectedly well, it might be continued as necessary after therapy has ceased, perhaps between long-term follow-ups, to take care of the occasional acute episode *of the same condition*. (The emphasis is necessary if a proving is to be avoided.)

2. If the similimum (or indeed the leading isopathic) was the patient's constitutional remedy, the patient may benefit from occasional dosing post-treatment. (However, note that the constitutional remedy may cause underlying conditions to come to the surface, necessitating further treatment.)

KEY CONCEPTS

Minimality theorem A disturbance of the life force will be annihilated by precisely the quantum of medicine that will cause the life force to resume its expression of the disturbance.

Posoequivalence theorem A single disturbance of the life force will call for a single dose of the medicine that will initiate cure.

Collective dose A dose of a given potentialised medicine, when dispensed as a set of exposures.

Split dose A dose of a homoeopathic medicine that anticipates an interruption, for example, sleep. It is given before and after the interruption.

Part 4 Homoeotherapy

9 The Clinical Approach

Introduction

What may be achieved?

We begin by asking what has brought the patient (or his parent) to the homoeopath. There will be at least one of the following reasons:

- the patient has a new comorbidity, unrelated to his autism
- the patient's autistic comorbidity seems to be worse

- the patient's primary autism seems to be more pronounced.

What should the practitioner aim for?

In the first case, the practitioner will naturally aim for a total resolution of the new problem, remembering that autistic people have a tendency to certain types of physical disorder, for example, autoimmune and gastrointestinal disorders.

In the second case the practitioner will be aim for a palliation of the problem, and search for the cause of the exacerbation.

In the third case, the practitioner will search for the exacerbating factor or modality, knowing that this could be a case of acute disease, for example, a new stress, or the signs of a prodrome. The practitioner's task will be made more difficult by the knowledge that palliation of the underlying or primary autism itself is not the aim (though a predisposition to anxiety will be a factor).

The autistic parent

The parent of the autistic patient will be desperate for a solution, but may well also be in need of assistance herself – for anxiety. (Also, she may be autistic too.)

The autistic patient

As for autism itself, I have assumed that the presenting complaint is a complication of an acute anxiety state of either known or unknown aetiology. I am unconvinced that an autistic anxiety state can be totally and permanently dispelled, but I have seen it respond positively to homoeopathy. Anxiety is always present in autism, and is easily precipitated or worsened by the slightest irritation or homoeopathic aggravation.

Naturally, the patient will as a matter of course be in need of bowel restoration, and will therefore require detoxification and dietary reconstruction. This is not optional if continued well-being is to be achieved.

Patients who are unaware of their autism

You will meet many patients who are completely unaware of their autism, and may consult you in relation to some other complaint. They will all be anxious – that is, as far as I am concerned, the keynote for the autistic patient – and may require treatment for that. However, aside from that, there is no need to introduce that new knowledge (it may only be your theory, of course) gratuitously.

Besides, an autistic patient who is at least middle aged will have figured out how to get by using unconscious avoidance and masking, and doing what he knows he likes. It is the young people, who are still in the thick of social turmoil, who have the most confusing lives.

The autistic practitioner

I have said that autistics make good homoeopaths. In fact, they are attracted to its system and rigour, its logical beauty and, of course, its books. For the author, homoeopathy was, and continues to be, in autistic parlance, a special interest.

A note on miasms in relation to autism

In the introduction to the *Homoeopathy 2.0* series of books, I wrote that one of my main concerns as a teacher was the general lack of understanding of the role of homoeopathy in the special areas of detoxification (sometimes called drainage), miasmic prescribing, and prophylaxis.

On contemplating this matter, I was led to the conclusion that, while *all* of the principles of homoeopathy in relation to cure could be derived from observations of the action of the similimum, *none* of them could logically be derived from the success of treatment strategies designed to relieve problems in these special areas.

Further enquiry showed me that the common factor among patients in these areas was a strong correlation with epidemic groups. This is a correlation that respondents to the similimum do not possess, and which their cure is independent of.

The principles of homoeopathy as enunciated in Book 1, Chapter 12: *Principles of Homoeopathic Medicine,* therefore do not have application to the treatment of a certain set of individuals: the members of *pathological groups*. The treatment of such patients is always designed either to eliminate a disorder of a group (classical: *miasm*) or (in the case of prophylaxis) to assuage an *anticipated* group disease.[7]

---

[7] The dynamics of group disease was introduced in Twohig, P 2021, *Case Management as a Clinical Technology,* Warburton Press Wyoming NSW, while its clinical solutions are outlined in Twohig, P 2021, *Introduction to Isopathic Prescribing,* Warburton Press Wyoming NSW.

Homoeopathic Solutions

The strategic approach

We need a strategic approach to autism, not least because the patient, especially if he is child, may not be forthcoming about his problems. In any case, there will be a history of some or all of the following:

- allopathic drug therapy
- family illness
- iatrogenic disease, e.g., from vaccination
- previous chronic disease
- suppression of typical childhood illness.

Typically, the patient may not be able to remember a time when he was well, no matter how old he is. The outmoded idea of treating 'layers' will not work with the autistic patient, not least because it assumes that the patient had a 'normal' layer to begin with, when he never did.

The neurodivergent response

The neurodivergent will respond to homoeopathy – wonderfully, in fact – however the practitioner may have to sacrifice some of his cherished ideas about the vital force to see the patient improve. What he will see in front of him is not a case of simple illness, but a case of illness being expressed by a uniquely autistic human: that is a challenge, because homeopathic technology is cliche-oriented.

The challenge lies in the patient's uniqueness. Simply put, there is no such thing as standard autism. Standard autism is a popular myth, one which the autistic people of the world are beginning to publicly decry in an effort to be accepted. Just as with a neurotypical patient, the autistic patient is responding to a disturbance of the vital force, one which is recognised, for example, toxicity, infection, etc.

However, he is not *simply* responding: his response will be compounded by a level of anxiety which may not be imaginable. He is not simply irritated at being ill, but also but by the totality of his responses, for which he has no solution. If he is a child he will have betrayed his illness by a complexity of clinical signs and somewhat automatic physical and mental signs known as stims (repetitive self-stimulating behaviour, for example, hand movements), the purpose of which is to relieve stress.

Removal of toxins (the isopathic approach)

It is safe to assume that the patient has been affected by the presence of toxins. I mentioned this in chapter 3 when discussing the universality of pseudochronic disease in autism, and the need to address it as a priority. I mentioned the means for its removal in introducing the eliminative mode of potencies, above.

The elimination of toxins should be considered as an introductory therapy, either alone or, if acute symptoms are present, alongside homoeopathy. The practitioner may also find it convenient to refer the patient to a physician who specialises in dietary advice *and* who is expert in the treatment of autistic people.

In any case, I will return to the subject of prescribing for the purpose of detoxification in chapter 11, as it involves simultaneous prescribing of potencies.

The leading remedy

In the case of a neurotypical patient, I would not advise leading with a partially palliative remedy, simply because the similimum will work more completely, and should therefore be the primary aim of case taking.

However, the autistic patient is often in need of rapid help, and that is best achieved by an *approximation* of the similimum, one that is known to work well in acute scenarios. A well-selected palliative may work instantly, giving the patient instant relief from his anxiety or illness. Indeed, the palliative may, if selected wisely, also turn out to be the curative. Recommended homoeopathic solutions to autistic anxiety are given in chapter 13.

Patient awareness

Since very few autistic adults are aware of their special neurodivergence, such patients will present with what they imagine is an entirely typical affliction (unless they have been referred), and may be treated as neurotypicals. If the patient is openly aware of his autism it will be easier to diagnose his presenting problem.

In the case of the autistic child, the parent may already be aware of the child's autism, and be able to discuss it. However, the practitioner must inform the parent that the child is not suffering from a medical disorder simply by reason of his autism, and make enquiry into the presenting problem, for example, ADHD.

It must always be remembered that the autistic patient will be constantly suffering from anxiety – that is his normal operating state.

Constitutional therapy

I have reserved a discussion of constitutional therapy for a later chapter, simply because this is one of the main areas of confusion in homoeopathy; yet it is one of the most noteworthy, and needs to be removed from the usual therapeutic discussion.

Miasmic treatment

We need to be clear that miasmic therapy is an isopathic protocol, and is therefore not curative. Miasmic therapy is the prescription of the miasm in potency, in the belief that it will eliminate the patient's dominant miasms or, in acute cases, the miasm governing the acute disease.

Regardless of the clinical presentation, the administration of a potentised remedy will not remove the patient's autism, though it might assuage his acute disease symptoms, especially if is caused by a microorganism.

10 Taking the Neurodivergent Case

Introduction

Taking the case of child if often impossible without most of the input coming from the parent. You should therefore take the case straight away, and assume that you will have all the information you need. Do not use questionnaires: the patient and the parent are sick of them Also, do not use a computer: it not you who is supposed to be the autistic (even if you are).

Case taking advice has been kept to a minimum except where it might be especially relevant to the autistic patient, as it assumed that the reader is either an advanced student or a professional homoeopath. That said, I would like to point out that this subject has been covered in depth in the three volumes comprising the *Homoeopathy 2.0* series of books,[8] in particular Book 2: *A Wholistic Approach to Homoeopathic Medicine* (2021).

The child

If you have an extroverted child who wants to speak, then you are in luck. you will be able to take the case easily, despite the fact that he might be restless, and might not sit down – he may even lie on the floor, pace, or hide behind something. He might also stim wildly (see below), be hyper-excited or speak loudly (as his normal state). (A word of caution: such a patient may know more about autism than you do.)

[8] A detailed description may be found at the end of this book.

However, if you have an in introverted child, especially one cannot speak, who is afraid of the clinical experience and of you, then your main informant will be the parent.

Special needs of the patient during the consultation

The parent may be asked before or during the consultation if there is anything that will help the child patient put up with the stress of the clinical experience. The patient may wish to bring a toy, stimming object or security object, for example, blanket along. He may also wish to eat or drink during the consultation. Even autistic adults have security objects and stimming toys – you can now buy them online – and if they have made an appointment to consult you about their autism, they might wish to bring them along.

The adult

The adult autistic patient who is aware of his comorbidity – though not necessarily his autism – will be a frank and reliable witness. ADHD is the most common comorbidity to autism, and remedies are not hard to find. As for autism itself, I have never treated an adult who desired a cure for his autism. The fact is that, in the experience of the author autistic people (including the author himself) would prefer to remain the way they are – comorbidities always excepted of course.

The homoeopathic solution for autistic anxiety uncomplicated by comorbidities is in itself not difficult to come up with.

Stimming

The autistic patient will be stimming during the consultation, either obviously, for example, swinging his leg, or in some way that is difficult to see, for example, clenching his toes. Whatever the case, you may be sure that he will need to stim even more once he is free to, owing to the stress of being observed and interrogated.

Stimming is a normal practice for the autistic, just as it is for the neurotypical. The difference lies in the constancy, intensity and variation. An autistic child, in particular, will likely be unable to exercise control over it (unless he has been disciplined for it).

It is worth mentioning that the autistic child will often self-harm if he is punished for stimming. Self-harming is far more common in girls, and may continue into adulthood. Self-harming is itself a form of stimming.

The myth of the autistic spectrum

It might be assumed that selecting the similimum for an autistic patient must be comparatively simply, as autistic people generally resemble each other, or because their presenting complaints are similar. However, both assumptions would be wrong. Autistic patients present with the same medical complaints as neurotypical patients, and in that respect are typical.

However, there exists a spectrum of nonphysical – one might say internal – differences that could describe the autistic individual's experience, a spectrum which differs from one individual to another, rendering the autistic person unique in a way that cannot be grokked by the neurotypical person, being a gestalt. This use of the term spectrum is not to be confused with the term commonly used by the ignorant and misinformed to describe autism as if it was comparable to a rainbow: the 'autistic spectrum'. The autistic spectrum in common parlance does not exist. Thus, an autistic is not 'on the spectrum' and does not 'suffer from ASD'.

Communication Issues

Masking

In the clinic masking will have an effect on the case as a whole, as the autistic patient is accustomed to mask whenever he is abroad, and especially when he aware that he is being observed. The purpose of masking is to 'pass' for neurotypical, which is something of a game for most autistics.

The simplest way to see if the patient is masking is to ask about it. You will, if the patient, permits, get a much clearer picture of his anxiety.

Be aware that females are so good at masking that it may be impossible to tell that they are autistic unless you are told. After all, it is normal for girls to socialise, and to want to seem friendly. Boys often do not care about such matters. Men will therefore be more open.

The pre-masking phase: children

Until they learn to mask, as they inevitably will, children will display their autism through neurodivergent behaviour. But gradually they will begin to copy their peers, though they will never entirely lose their autistic behaviour, especially when alone.

Masking in adolescents

Most girls will learn to pass for neurotypical in their early teens. However, most boys will never truly master the art, and will wind up getting labelled as 'geeks' and 'nerds', especially if they display high intelligence.

Masking in adults

Adult masking is usually complete: the adult patient is typically a parent and spouse, with a job and financial responsibilities. He has therefore learned the art of getting on with people, and is highly unlikely to throw all that away because he feels like stimming in front of his peers. Instead, he is apt to drink, take drugs, and be violent in private.

Adults most at risk of betraying their autism are therefore epileptics. The author has known many, and is himself one, and what saves them from *complete and permanent* shunning is the popular belief that they are suffering from a medical condition, which is not the same as a neurodivergence, you will notice.

The patient's frame of mind

The autistic detests attempts at sincerity, and abhors small talk or polite conversation (and there is very good chance that his parent is the same).

To the extent that the patient understands and accepts his condition, on the other hand he may be happy to be share his interesting life with you, and in fact might be extremely loquacious. Many autistics are quite happy to find that they are in some way special, gifted or interesting people, and many of them actually make autism a special interest (and hence this book).

The autistic patient may be unable or unwilling to smile, and may maintain a 'plain face'. He may not appreciate attempts at humour. Also, he will take everything he hears literally.

If he asks a question, he will expect an honest and professional answer. He will only ask a question if he wants to know the answer: he is not interested in being polite, and may appear rude.

How to communicate

The way to communicate is sincerely and with eye contact (without expecting the patient to reciprocate: quite simply, he will find eye contact painful). The practitioner's voice should be gentle and his questions reasonable, because the autistic is above all logical and may be humourless (think Mr Spock from Star Trek – though he is not an autistic: he is a Vulcan, which is a different thing altogether).

If you patronise the autistic you will instantly lose his respect and he may cease to cooperate. Given that your patient is used to being patronised but not happy about it, you may have an uphill battle trying to regain his confidence.

Finally, it may be extremely unwise to actually touch your autistic patient, unless he decides to, for example, extent a hand. Autistics are pathologically clean people and often assume that everyone else is a potential contaminant (think Young Sheldon).

Barriers to taking the family history

The practitioner should take a family history of occurrences of neurodivergence and possible comorbidities, including epilepsy, bowel disorder and autoimmune disease.

The following are common impediments to obtaining a reliable family history:

- alcoholism
- deceased parent
- either parent is adopted
- a history of incorrect diagnoses
- secrecy concerning these or similar conditions within the family.

Clinical Signs and Symptoms

Autism and autistic anxiety

I have included the following list as likely signs and symptoms that will be observed by and reported to the practitioner. Some will be worse for stress, which is why they are listed.

Burnout, exhaustion, reduced action
Carbohydrates, craves
Communication skills lacking; may not pick up on facial expressions or body language
Compulsion to do what he wants to do
Crying, excessive

Dairy products, craves
Echolalia: may respond to questions by automatically repeating the question
Feeding problems
Fussiness, especially about rules, placement of objects, correctness
Hyperactive
Lack of eye contact
Lack of socials skills, especially emotional reciprocity
Meltdowns
Oversensitivity to environmental stimuli such as sounds and light and clothing
Paces constantly
Photosensitivity, and other over-sensitivities
Regression, in response to vaccination. The child may also lose the power of speech, which Regression, loss of power of speech
Regression, spontaneous
Regression, stops smiling.
Repetitive actions, especially hand-flapping and speech
Response to name absent
Restless
Sensory issues: everything too strong, overwhelming
Shut-downs
Sleep issues, can only sleep for short periods
Smiles, does not
Social interaction, avoids
Speech delay
Speech issues: babbles meaninglessly; screeches

Stimming
Sweets, craves
Toilet training problems
Vaccination, autism worse for
Violent sudden body movements

Comorbidities

ADD

Absent-minded, mentally dull and sluggish
Inattention
Daydreaming excessively
Easily distracted

ADHD

Aggression, irritability, tantrums
Hyperactivity
Restlessness and fidgeting
Explosive energy
Lack of concentration
Problems following instructions
Has trouble completing tasks
Doesn't listen
Is a messy worker
Talks too much
Clumsy
Loses things
Is easily bored
Impulsivity

- *Alexithymia* – Inability to identify his emotions

- *Anxiety* – While that is technically a comorbidity, most autistics are clinically anxious.
- *Bowel problems, constipation, diarrhoea* – Leaky gut syndrome is extremely common in autism and its comorbidities, due to dietary problems (See Appendix 1)
- *Depression*
- *Dyscalculia* – Difficulty performing arithmetic and mathematical calculations
- *Dysgraphia* – Difficulty writing due to lack of fine motor skills
- *Dyslexia* – Difficulty understanding words and letters, (a common comorbidity of ADHD)
- *Dyspraxia* – Difficulty in coordination, resulting in clumsiness, lack or fine or gross motor control, affecting 5-6 per cent of school-age children (and, therefore, adults). Examples of fine motor control problems are: using a knife and fork, gripping pencils correctly, doing up shoe laces, shaving, applying make-up. Examples of gross motor problems are: dropping things, tripping over, learning to drive (many autistics and dyspraxics don't drive), ambidexterity, and difficulty telling right from left. Proprioception spatial awareness) problems. Also, *verbal dyspraxia* (see below).
- *Epilepsy* – Seizure disorder is the most common autistic comorbidity. Perhaps 39% of autistics suffer from seizure disorder. Homoeopathically, Cannabis Indica may be particularly useful. Cannabidiol supplementation and a ketogenic diet have also been found useful at reducing seizures.

- *Gastrointestinal disorders* – Most autistics have inflammatory bowel disease, constipation, diarrhoea, reflux, and food allergies. All of these problems have been linked to gut dysbiosis. Because some gut proteins and microbial products can enter the bloodstream and cross the blood-brain barrier, mast cells can be activated, resulting in a cycle of chronic inflammation.
- *Intellectual disability* – Approximately half of autistics have some degree of intellectual disability.
- *Learning disability* – Approximately half of autistics have a learning disability.
- *Sensory processing disorder* – Most autistics have an oversensitivity or undersensitivity to physical stimuli, including pain. No sensory type is excluded. Thus, for example, the patient, especially if a child, may not be able to tolerate the sensation of certain foods in his mouth, or certain colours, shapes or noises. He may have temperature oversensitivity, and prefer very hot or very cold environments. He may always wear sunglasses when he is outside, and avoid noise.
- *Verbal dyspraxia* – Speech and language impairment, especially difficulty making speech sounds and forming sentences.
- *Working memory disorder* – This is a problem often seen in dyspraxics, and relates to day to day memory problems, for example, losing things. Memory impairment may affect patients' abilities to learn, despite strong language skills.

Case Analysis

Aim

The central questions of the case

Usually when we see a new patient, especially a child with a puzzling presentation, we are full of questions about aetiology. However, when the child's mother says there is a history of autism, we only need to consider a few aetiological question. That is because we already know that the child has always been autistic, and always will be. It is his current suffering (and that of the parent) we wish to allay.

However, the purpose of those questions is:

- to ascertain what may be healed (palliated)
- to ascertain what factors, if any, have historically contributed to the patient's condition
- to ascertain the obstacles to cure.

In the last chapter we discussed the likely signs and symptoms of the autistic child, especially when anxious, and especially when there are comorbidities. The practitioner will therefore have a guide to the child's likely make-up and habits – the parent will fill in the gaps.

The secondary questions

Throughout the consultation, we bear in mind what we know about autism, all the while asking the questions needed to ascertain the set of rubrics we will be constructing, including modalities.

Usually when taking the case, the practitioner might ask questions in a certain order that he is used to. By all means continue to do this. However, be mindful of the time constraint involved: neither the parent nor the patient will be at ease in your presence, and the patient may have little patience. Thus, as soon as you can get to the heart of the problem, do not hesitate to prescribe.

You will find it a simple matter to take the case if you remember that you do not need to 'cure' the patient's many comorbidities, nor to dispel his autism, nor to work out his constitutional remedy. For that reason, I have kept case taking to a minimum. Remember that you will never see two autistics who are alike.

Strategic questions

In order to develop a clinical strategy, the practitioner will need to consider:

- what is the main disturbance of the life force
- what must he palliated and in what order
- what is actually incurable
- what are the obstacles to cure.

The treatment support strategy

In order to develop a clinical support strategy, the practitioner will need to consider:

- to what extent cure is being held up by environmental toxicity
- the best way to eliminate toxicity
- the supportive measures, if any, to be prescribed.

Modalities

Normally, we place great stock in modalities. With the autistic you will find that there may well be so many (especially *worse for*) that you are overwhelmed. By all means look for leading modalities, but do not be surprised if this approach fails, especially because the modality may not be in the Repertory.

Findings

For the patient record

For the patient's record you might make a note of:

- leading problems and symptoms apart from the usual neurodivergences
- any evidence or record of toxicity
- evidence of bowel disorder
- any notable features of the patient's diet.

The constitutional remedy

During the course of case taking, you will have intuited the patient's notional constitutional remedy. Simply make a note of it for future reference. It may or may not be the similimum on that particular day. The constitutional diathesis may be obvious: the Calc. cliche, the Phos. cliche, the Tub. cliche, etc. But this is no time to be heroic. (See also chapter 13)

Potency selection and posology

Questions relating to potency selection and posology were discussed in chapters 7-8.

Primary remedy candidates

List the main remedies to be considered, and record the homoeopathic and isopathic solutions, including advice given to the parent, especially on now to administer medicines and judge their effects. For example,

For anxiety:

Vaccininum 1M once a week

Sil. 1LM every 4 hours (plussed) until >

For bowel dysbiosis:

Candida 1M + Lyc. 24C

am and pm until >.

11 First Prescription & Review

First Prescription

Instructions to the patient

Homoeopathic instructions

The patient will need clear instructions concerning the administration of the medicines, and what to expect, if anything. She should also be given clear directions for plussing, and for *extended divided dosing*, if the patient is extremely sensitive, and bearing in mind that he will almost have hypersensitivities as yet unseen.

The patient may be unaware of the nature of autism, and have been exposed to a lot of different opinions, some of them medical She will therefore need to be assured that the condition itself is neither rare nor pathological, simply extremely trying for those who don't understand it.

The patient should be instructed not to take allopathic medicine designed to suppress the common signs of the presenting complaint, unless absolutely necessary, excluding anti-epileptic drugs, of course. If she finds it necessary to suppress, for example rage, then dosing will have to be restarted.

Detoxification instructions

It will be necessary to have a conversation about what may need to be done to support the patient in the area of diet, as outlined in Appendix 1. You might wish to make up a hand-out to assist her.

Common sources of toxins

In addition, you might wish to include in your hand-out a list of the most common toxins to avoid, which is even more relevant if your client is a woman who uses cosmetics. Some of the more common ones are:

- aluminium, (contained in many personal care products)
- cleaning products, especially those used around the house
- fluoride (present in tap water and most toothpastes)
- perfumes (autistics often cannot tolerate them in any form)
- sodium lauryl sulphate (present in shampoos, soaps and toothpastes)
- talc.

Dispensing the medicine

The parent should be told that the preferred way for the patient to take the medicine is to swallow it. If the patient is unable to swallow the medicine it may be given to him surreptitiously, perhaps in his food or drink. Basically, there is no limit to the ways in which potencies may be administered.

Remedy multiplicity

Concurrent medicines

Because the autistic presentation may have been muddied by:

- previous homoeopathic prescribing
- a history of allopathic drugs
- a history of vaccination
- a history of dietary abuse
- a history of chronic disease

you will find it necessary to prescribe concurrent remedies. Remember that this is perfectly acceptable, provided that you only prescribe:

- one similimum at a time, e.g., Stannum Metallicum
- one elimination remedy at a time, e.g., Vaccininum
- one support remedy at a time, e.g., Thuja.

Intercurrent remedy

If the patient is a child with a special need, for example, a remedy for screaming only, you might want to prescribe such a remedy, for example, Apis 30C, to be kept on hand by the parent. That remedy might turn out to be worth its weight in gold.

Prescription Writing

It is important that you keep a clear and complete record of everything that was done in the consultation, in case you have to refer to the patient to another homoeopathic physician. In particular, may have noted something about the patient that he might miss.

Review Arrangement

It will be necessary to review the patient eventually, as there will be much work to be done by way of monitoring his progress, especially in the light necessary dietary changes.

Follow-up & Second Prescription

Follow-up consultation

Initial questions

Autistic patients, particularly children, may be difficult to monitor, so you need to ascertain whether the prescription was followed, and, if not, the reason. Initially, ask:

- Did the patient take the medicine?
- How did he take the medicine?
- When did he take the medicine?
- What happened when he took the medicine?
- Has he taken any other therapeutic measures?

The answers to these questions may be all you need to prescribe a second time.

Case taking questions

For a neurotypical patient, you may need to ask a lot of questions to take the case again. However, the autistic's parent is usually impatient to tell you how the remedy went, one way or another. The main topic you will want to pursue is aggravation.

Clinical Aggravation

I am going to discuss *aggravation* first up, as it can be alarming. While the practitioner should not deliberately attempt to induce it, he should never be surprised when it appears in an autistic patient.

Homoeopathic aggravation

There are two types of aggravation: homoeopathic and isopathic. In the first case, we see a more or less worsening of the leading symptoms following the administration of the similimum. If the aggravation is not great, we need do nothing, knowing that the healing gradient has been correctly installed and that eventually the aggravation will pass and be followed by a general amelioration.

If the aggravation is great, on the other hand, we may need to antidote the symptoms being displayed by the patient. If the symptoms are not new, we will know what to do, because we will have anticipated such an event. When dealing with autistics, anticipation is essential.

Antidoting

It is important to note that you must not antidote *the remedy*. An antidote does not antidote a remedy but a *remedy response*. Thus, if you do not understand the nature of the response you must see the patient again. You may use an internet connection for that purpose. Also, an antidote must not be based on rule of thumb, but on repertorisation.

Remember that if you successfully antidote a remedy response, the symptom picture will return to its previous state. Eventually, therefore, you will have to prescribe again, possibly the remedy that you had to antidote if in a lower potency.

Isopathic aggravation

In the second case we see a great aggravation from an isopathic remedy. There are two kinds of isopathic remedies:

those that have been proved and those that have not. As isopathics are given to eliminate toxins and group disease vectors, most of them have not been proved. An accidental proving of such a remedy will look like a general (and generally slight) aggravation of the patient's pre-existing symptoms (because he is already suffering from toxicity due to the substance or influence from which it was made). As you will have anticipated such a response with the appropriate homoeopathic supportive or palliative, this should not be problematic.

On the other hand, an isopathic that has been made from a proven homoeopathic remedy, for example, Vaccininum, will give an aggravation in line with its materia medica entry, and a proving of such a remedy will present *new* symptoms which will be in line with that entry, so you will be able to see what has happened. Note that a proving is an indication that you have greatly underestimated the patient's sensitivity, and probably the medicine's power. If you do nothing the symptoms will abate.

Constitutional aggravation

A constitutional aggravation is a homoeopathic aggravation following the administration of a similimum that is also the patient's constitutional remedy – they are not necessarily the same thing. Such a remedy can have strong and lasting benefits, though that is not advanced as a recommendation. Each remedy has its right time.

The healing response

Let me remind you that the autistic healing response is not like the response of the patient who has chronic disease: steady, stepwise, retrogression leading to health (allowing for age, etc.). The autistic is suffering from the results of both exogenous stress and endogenous stress, usually due to poor diet, which must be reduced and attended to, respectively. His healing will take time, and will never result in the removal of his autism (or his neurological comorbidities), but might be on level that is incomprehensible to the neurotypical.

The order of healing

The order in which healing occurs is determined by the *order of healing theorem,* which predicts that, as healing progresses, pathology will retrogress; and the *healing characteristics theorem,* which predicts that radiant healing will occur with the characteristics of the life force.

The first theorem in effect predicts that the patient will instantaneously be aware that healing is taking place, without being able to identify the change. The second predicts that the patient will experience certain events, e.g thriving, freeing up of function, more effective communication, improved relationship, and improved communication, not to mention well-being.

Naturally, the autistic probably won't mention the first type of change, but he will display at least some of the characteristics of the second kind. Simply put, if he was previously unhappy and stressed out, he might be better, which is saying a lot.

Amelioration

If amelioration is partial and not complete, this is to be expected in a case with perhaps numerous comorbidities and underlying bowel dysbiosis. Further prescribing will no doubt result in further amelioration. On the other hand, if there is a significant general improvement which then subsides, it simply means that the healing gradient was not sufficient, and that further prescribing of the same remedy in a higher dosage and perhaps potency should be tried.

KEY CONCEPTS

Aggravation 1. Allopathic a. Iatrogenic poisoning. 2. **Homoeopathic a.** An acute transient episode of the presenting symptoms following homoeopathic medication. It is due to an apparent acceleration of the life force in the direction of the desuppression. 3. **Isopathic a**. An aggravation of symptoms following the administration of an isopathic medicine. It is due to a proving of the vector. 4. **Constitutional a.** Transient symptomatic amplification following administration of the constitutional remedy.

Healing characteristics theorem Radiant healing occurs with the characteristics of the life force.

Order of healing theorem As healing progresses pathology retrogresses.

12 Constitutional Prescribing

Introduction

The subjects of the constitution and the constitutional remedy need to be discussed in a special chapter because:

- the nature of the constitution and diathesis need to be explained
- the special role of the constitutional remedy in therapy needs to be explained

- the constitutional remedy is often wrongly prescribed as if it was always the similimum
- the incorrect prescription of the constitutional remedy can result in a disordered case.

As well as examining these matters, we will consider the likelihood that the autistic diathesis is actually the result of an identifiable constitution, having a family of distinct remedy relationships. If that is the case, it might greatly simply the selection of remedies.

Finally, we will look at the proper use of the constitutional remedy in autistic presentations, because it is not as straightforward as it might be in neurotypical presentations.

Constitution and Diathesis

What is the constitution?

There is an enormous confusion in homoeopathy about the nature of the constitution and its signature remedy, the constitutional. I have addressed these matters in depth in *A Vitalistic Approach to Homoeopathy*. In this book, I will simply summarise what the practitioner may need to know when treating the autistic patient.

The constitution is a theoretical construct of all that may be pathological in the individual: in that sense it is pure potentiality. Therefore, it may be thought of as being the sum of all the patient's susceptibilities in every vital sphere and the source of any spontaneous illness. Naturally, it includes his susceptibilities to homoeopathic remedies, especially when we consider that a homoeopathic medicine once taken becomes a *disturbance*.

Speaking clinically, we say that the constitution represents:

- the consequences of unresolved disease
- environmental influences that have been inherited one way or another
- unresolved pathophysiological problems from earlier generations.

The latter appear in the form of congenital *differences*, that is, pathophysiologies stripped of their pathologies but not their physiognomies or peculiarities. These may be transmitted genetically, and one can't help wondering if they are connected to the phenomenon of neurodivergence, especially as neither the constitution nor the autistic phenomenon is a disease state.

The function of the constitution is to provide an individuating indicator of the lifelong healing journey of the human which began at conception.

What is the diathesis?

Thus, the constitution displays the diathesis or pathophysiological typology of the patient, that is, the set of features and characteristic that, from the homoeopathic point of view invariably indicate a family of remedies which will be found to include the constitutional remedy itself.

The diathesis is the distinctive physiology of the patient. It comprises the minute differences that give rise to the remedies and of course the rubrics that point to them. Despite the fact that the constitutional diathesis is a distinctly clinical phenomenon, it is not something that needs to be resolved, like a disease.

Thus, we may speak of the 'tubercular diathesis', the 'autoimmune diathesis', and so on. Note that each of the diatheses indicates a genus of remedy. It might therefore be reasonable to posit the existence of an autistic diathesis.

Chapter 13 contains a list of homoeopathic remedies that I believe might be prime candidates for the treatment of autistic anxiety. These might be thought of as the group belonging to the autistic diathesis. The 'stamp' of the autistic diathesis, in its simplest terms, is the description given in chapter 1.

Remember that, because neither the diathesis nor the constitution that gives rise to it are total symptom pictures, they may not be prescribed to (though a comorbid overlay may), though we may treat the autistic patient's problems, for example, anxiety.

What is the constitutional remedy?

The constitutional remedy in relation to a given patient is the remedy which singularly is reminiscent of the constitution of the patient. When administered, it immediately amplifies the patient's constitution, including any divergences from the norm, pathological and physiological. Also:

- Were we to see new symptoms that the patient admits he had been experiencing but had not mentioned, that would give us a more complete symptom picture to prescribe to (using a different remedy).

- Were we to see a brief aggravation followed by amelioration we would need look no further for the similimum.
- Were we to see new symptoms that are characteristic of the remedy but not the patient, that would be evidence of a clinical proving, and might require antidoting to bring the true picture back.

The usefulness of the constitutional concept

There is no such thing in homoeopathy as the treatment of the constitution, simply because that entity is entirely theoretical, and has no foundation in the presenting pathophysiology. The concept is enormously useful, however, because it provides the vitalistic physician with his *sole* access point to the patient's vitalist nature.

The practitioner may well have his symptomatology and diagnostic signs, and his various tests. However, only through his realisation of the gestalt of the patient may he divine the similimum and its satellitium of related remedies, which are always indicated by of the constitution.

How the constitutional remedy relates to the patient

The constitutional remedy is not a homoeopathic for the patient: instead, it is isopathic to the patient's *diathesis*, that is, its presence causes the diathesis to attempt to eliminate inherited unresolved deep vitalistic pathophysiology, the kind that is only indicated by the patient's physicality and mentality, and is perhaps experienced in the form of chronic disorders that appear spontaneously during his life journey, for example, as spontaneous illnesses resulting from apparent predispositions.

The attempt to eliminate what may be the remnants of ancestral disease causes an expansion of the vital force, forcing any current disease overlay to be displayed. What we see could well be the similimum; however, other related remedies might also appear, giving us a group to choose from.

The constitutional remedy is only homoeopathic in that its presence causes the patient's resonance with the morphic field of the disease to be weakened. However, the constitutional remedy is always identified with a homoeopathic remedy, and just as often performs as the similimum.

Why is that? The fact is that the set of similar and related remedies that constitute the *diathetical group* always contains one remedy that acts as the generic similimum, regardless of what we may call it. The emergence of the diathetical group is a response to the presentation itself, and gives rise to the short-listed remedies.

The Autistic Constitution

The autistic constitution and the neurodivergent diathesis

The autistic constitution

Given that a constitution is a theoretical homoeopathic type, how may we construct a typology for the autistic? First, we take the main, that is, generally agreed upon, 'symptoms' (from chapter 1):

'Symptomatology'

- Deficiency in social/emotional reciprocity (the give and take of social intercourse)
- A lack of nonverbal communication, including eye contact and gestures
- Difficulty in the area of relationships, including their development, maintenance and understanding of them
- Repetitive speech, body movements or movement of an object
- Insistence on sameness
- An intense special interest
- Hypersensitivities

Characteristics

He arranges, organises, and creates beats and rhythms, repeatable programmes, cyclic events and crystalline conceptuals and sets. He is a musician, collector, regular sufferer, pattern-maker, rule-maker, legislator, designer, architect, mathematician, programmer, inventor and game player.

Key characteristic

The key characteristic is iteration/rhythmicity/crystallinity.

Generic isopathic

The constitution is always based on an isopathic generic typology, for example, tuberculosis, carcinosis, etc. without presupposing a causal relationship. In this case let us refer to prototypical isopathic as Vaccininum – again, no cause is presupposed.

Remedy family candidates

The next step is to derive from the emergent typology a possible family of remedies. Prime candidates might be:

Alumina
Alumina Silicata
Antimonium Tartaricum
Apis
Baryta Carbonica
Calcarea Carbonica
Calcarea Silicata
Cannabis Indica
Carcinosinum
Cuprum Aceticum
Cuprum Metallicum
Ferrum Phosphoricum
Fluoricum Acidum
Granite
Histaminum
Kali Bromatum
Kali Cyanatum
Kali Muriaticum
Luna
Lycopodium
Lyssinum
Magnesia Carbonica
Phosphorus
Silica
Thuja

Zincum Metallicum

Provisional Remedy 'family'

Alumina Silicata
Calcarea Silicata
Granite
Kali Muriaticum
Luna
Silica

Remedy representative of family

Let us say that the typifying, that is, prototypical, remedy is Silica.

Of course, it may be that this whole procedure is amiss, but it's a beginning. In chapter 13 I suggest a longer list of possible remedies to consider for autistic anxiety, and many of these remedies are also suggestive of the symptoms of autistic comorbidities.

I am not suggesting that every autistic patient will exactly fit this typology. I myself have never needed any of the remedies on the above short list, and only taken one on the long list, despite having taken many remedies.

The neurodivergent diathesis

Now it is possible to see, looking at the above list, and group, how we are merely prescribing to an entity that is derivative, regardless of the symptom picture. All the indicators we need to prescribe are given to us by the neurodivergent diathesis, which might in the case of the individual be unique. That is why we need to take the case carefully.

Prescribing Issues

General constitutional issues

In chapter 6 I discussed the modes in which potencies may be observed to operate. After all, the constitutional is a remedy, and as such operates in every dynamic mode. However, when the constitutional is pressed into service for the wrong reason, that is, in the wrong mode, not only will it not achieve the desired effect, its action may seem paradoxical.

For example, the practitioner might realise early in the consultation that he is looking at a Causticum type (the Causticum *cliche*, so to speak) and proceed to prescribe that remedy, confident that it must be the similimum for 'the patient', who is thought to be 'suffering from autism'. Full of confidence, he prescribes Causticum 10M, which happens to be the constitutional.

He does not realise that the patient's autism is not a curable condition, and that he has not therefore correctly diagnosed the presenting complaint or remedy. The result is an inexplicable aggravation on a scale commensurate with the power of the medicine. That is because the function of the constitutional remedy is to sensitise the patient to his own constitution.

As another example, the practitioner picks up on the Causticum, but belongs to the school that whatever he observes must be the patient's constitution, and that the constitutional remedy and the similimum are the same thing, and that he must please the parent by prescribing Causticum 10M. The result is the same as in first example.

A third example. The practitioner painstakingly takes the case and listens to everything the parent says. However, he can't help observing that the patient is happy and outgoing, talkative, looks him in the eye with wide, bright eyes, and is polite. The mother reports that she is the best student in her class. For him, that is enough. He prescribes Phosphorus 1M (though he does not see what all the fuss is about), and sends them away. He completely discounts what the mother says about her daughter's behaviour at home: stimming, screaming, and the like, because he does not understand autism. What he has been observing is *masking*, which *all* autistics engage in all their lives. When the patient gets home, she experiences a meltdown. She never takes the remedy.

Issues in autistic presentations

However, the autistic does not present as a standard autistic human, and may appear to be completely different to every autistic you have heard about. You must therefore take his word, or his parent's, that he is autistic, and that he has this or that comorbidity or medical problem. Most of the autistics I have met did display at least some neurodivergent characteristics, but apart from the children, all of them had learned to mask, some perfectly.

You must bear in mind at all times that autism is essentially an interior condition, and that the so-called autistic spectrum is an inner one, completely different for each individual, and invisible to the outer world.

However, the main message here is that, unless your patient does not mention being autistic, your will take the case as you normally would, in the knowledge that the correct remedy is always the similimum.

Leading with the patient's constitutional remedy

I should caution the practitioner: a constitutional remedy when prescribed as such will have the effect of amplifying the homoeopathic constitution anywhere from a little to a lot, which in turn will amplify any presenting complaints and autistic comorbidities.

This side-effect has the advantage of throwing the symptom picture into relief, thus facilitating remedy diagnosis, and the disadvantage of amplifying symptoms which might interfere with case taking, for example, hyperactivity.

That said, the possibility of the constitutional remedy is that it will have an ameliorative effect, though that is not to be expected and might only occur when the presenting symptoms have been artificially amplified by some other intervening factor (which may not have a physical presence, for example, psychological trauma).

Generally, the constitutional will not be the similimum for the overlay that constitutes the presenting problem: that work will be performed by the curative or by several palliatives, for example, similimums. Thus, the practitioner might know perfectly well what the constitutional is, but may never need to prescribe it.

Because this caution cannot be overstressed I give the following example. The patient, an autistic child, presents with a Chamomilla constitution. However, his acute complaint is bronchitis of recent origin. On the one hand, we think of Chamomilla; but then we learn that his characteristic irritability has been less since the onset of the bronchitis. On further investigation we decide to give Spongia, especially because the symptoms are < eating. There was no need to begin with the constitution, because the symptomatology was clear, as was the remedy.

When to prescribe the constitutional remedy

In the case of neurotypicals, the time to prescribe the constitutional remedy is when there is little or no symptom picture.

Let's be clear about this: the primary function of the constitutional remedy *as such*, is to produce symptoms: that is its action in the amplificational mode as mentioned in chapter 6. It is only when we see those symptoms that we search for the similimum (which might end up being the constitutional remedy itself).

If we do not observe anything to prescribe to – there could be any number of reasons for this situation, the most common in neurotypicals being deep pathology – the usual procedure is to give the constitutional remedy to produce a picture, and then prescribe the similimum for it. However, that is something we never do with autistics.

First, they are not inherently diseased: their reported presentation is their optimum operating state, whether we like it or not. Secondly, they may appear to be completely normal (making their parent look pretty foolish into the bargain) because of their genius for masking. Third – and in my experience, far more likely – they may be shut down or profoundly shy, or both. To be perfectly clear, if you prescribe a homoeopathic in any of these circumstances, you will produce a proving of the remedy, which could be disastrous.

When not to prescribe the constitutional remedy

In the clinic we observe symptoms. When they are present we prescribe the constitutional remedy only if it is also the similimum or a remedy we wish to use for amplification or in the eliminative mode, for example, Cannabis Sativa. In this regard, we should never think of the constitutional as a panacea: it is not that.

KEY CONCEPTS

Constitution The complete organism in all of its spheres: behavioural, intellectual, emotional, physical, being the sum of all that it has inherited and acquired.

Constitutional diathesis The features of a given constitution that leads it to be susceptible to specific morbific agents or influences and predisposed to specific forms of illness.

Constitutional prescribing Prescribing a remedy that matches the patient's apparent constitutional picture, for the purpose of amplifying the patient's vital force.

Constitutional, -al remedy A remedy that is reminiscent of the constitution of a patient.

Part 5 Special Materia Medica

Materia Medica

SILICA
STAPHYSAGRIA
STRAMONIUM
SULPHUR
TARENTULA HISPANICA
THUJA
TUBERCULINUM
VERATRUM ALBUM
ZINCUM METALLICUM

Introduction

The particular suitability of the homoeopathic materia medica

The particular suitability of the homoeopathic materia medica for the treatment of autistic patients lies in the fact that it does not contain pat solutions to the problems of autistics; put another way, it does not treat the autistic patient as a stereotype. That turns out to be a very handy thing, because every autistic person is uniquely neurodivergent, and therefore may be thought of as a human possessed of an additional experiential and existential dimension.

In fact, as I have stated elsewhere, I have often thought that autistics might be thought of as a separate human species We can therefore afford to be very choosy when it comes to repertorisation, safe in the knowledge that we are not trampling all over sacred medical definitions, and that is because autism per se is not a morbidity, despite being long thought of as one by the ignoramuses. The fact is that autistics are more often than not the bearers of morbidities whose symptoms may be found in the repertory, which facilitates searching.

Remedies for the autistic species

The problem facing the practitioner will be to distinguish what might be minimised, cured and so on. The autistic who is not aware of this problem will give far too much information, believing that the homoeopath, like all of the physicians he has ever seen, wants him to describe his autism. However, having said that, it is now necessary to say that the homoeopath does need to be able make distinctions.[9] He should therefore ensure that he defines the presenting problem. Usually, of course, he will be assisted in this task by a parent.[10]

In this book I have assumed that the presenting patient is autistic and may or may not have a common comorbidity. I have assumed that a person who has only *one* of the common autistic comorbidities probably does not exist. Neurodiversity is just that: diverse. Thus, in this chapter I have listed common autistic signs together with common comorbid symptoms when they feature in the remedy picture and when they

---

[9] After much experimentation I decided against including a rubric index, as the autistic presentation is not easy to repertorise. I am confident that the experienced practitioner will only need his knowledge of the remedy keynotes, and the following guide.

[10] I have preferred symptoms that you would expect to see in a child.

appear in the *Materia Medica* – I emphasise that, because usually they do not.[11][12]

I should say from the outset that I have only included a group of promising epilepsy remedies with the caveat that the epileptic patient must remain on anticonvulsant medication during treatment, and may therefore not benefit from any homoeopathic which is prescribed with epilepsy as a leading symptom. I say this as an epilepsy sufferer myself, one who has experimented and failed.

Isopathics

The practitioner will always be tempted to prescribe a group disease (classical: *miasm*) remedy for the autistic patient, in the belief that he is suffering from a group disease. There is a place for these remedies in isopathic therapy. Examples are: the vaccines, other nosodes, bacterial overgrowths, for example, Candida Albicans, and substances which are prescribed to eliminate toxins, for example, Plumbum Metallicum.

---

[11] Remedies I excluded from the short list (to save space) were: Alf., Allium-s., Arn., Ars., Aur-m., Bell., Calad., Calc-p., Camph., Cham., Cina, Coff., Con., Cupr-cy., Graph., Hyos., Ign., Kali-p., Merc., and Nat-m. I know that many of them (and others) will occur to the experienced practitioner, as appropriate.

[12] The *Materia Medica* used was Robin Murphy's *Lotus Materia Medica*.

ALUMINA

Characteristic symptoms

Sluggishness, and general fatigue, mainly after speaking.

Much trembling of the body as a whole.

Burning pain in lower back.

Characteristic mental symptoms

Confusion as to identity.

Constant moaning, fretting.

Hasty, hurried.

Sneers at everything.

Memory bad.

Everything viewed in bad light.

Hasty but executes slowly.

Makes mistakes writing and speaking.

Timorous.

Vague, reserved and unobserving.

Other useful symptoms

Ailments from anger.

> Open air.

< Potatoes, warmth, starch, speaking, full and new moon.

Taste disordered.

Aversion meat, potatoes.

Craves coarse food.

No desire to eat.

Staggers on walking.

ALUMINA SILICATA

Characteristic symptoms

The child will not be touched.

Marked constriction.

Epileptiform convulsions.

Brain disorders.

Pain in head > heat.

Limbs jerk.

Other useful symptoms

> Warmth, fasting, in bed.

< Eating, standing, evening.

Skin < touch, pressure.

ANTIMONIUM TARTARICUM

Characteristic symptoms

Children have convulsions if attention is thrust upon them.

Chronic trembling of head and hands.

Convulsive twitching.

Convulsions.

Cries during sleep with fixed eyes and trembling.

Characteristic mental symptoms

Child is wishes to be carried upright, and unwilling to be looked at or touched.

Effects of anger or vexation.

Ill-effects of vaccination.

Female: puerperal convulsions.

On falling asleep, electric-like shocks.

Child coughs when angry.

Useful general symptoms

Averse milk.

Thirstless.

Desires water little and often.

Desires apples, fruit and acids, which <.

APIS

Characteristic symptoms

Allergic response.

Ill effects of vaccination.

Causations: grief, rage fright, vexation, jealousy, bad news, mental shock.

Sudden shrill cries.

Extreme sensitiveness to the slightest touch.

Prostration even to faintness.

Characteristic mental symptoms

Fussy, fidgety, hard to please.

Fear of being poisoned.

Whines constantly.

Sudden shrill piercing screams.

Cries all day and all night.

Apathy and indifference.

Listless, cannot think clearly.

Cannot concentrate on reading and writing.

Nothing seems to satisfy.

Childish and silly behaviour in women after birth.

Useful general symptoms

> Cool air, cool bathing, uncovering, sitting erect.

< Any form of heat, hot drinks, bath, bed, pressure, touch.

Craves milk.

BARYTA CARBONICA

Characteristic symptoms

Children underdeveloped, dull, apathetic, averse to new people.

Prostration, weariness.

Paralytic condition.

Mistrust, want of self-confidence, averse to strangers.

Does not want to play.

Characteristic mental symptoms

Talks in sleep.

Sleepy and weary on slightest effort.

Anxious dreams, frequent waking.

Mistrustful.

Shy of strangers.

Forgets her errand or words in her mouth.

Lost confidence in himself.

Bashful, timid.

Cowardly.

Hides behind furniture.

Brain fog, confusion.

Idiocy. Low mental grasp.

Whining mood.

Silly, absurd.

Talking mania in menses in girls.

Does not want to play, but sits alone.

Child cannot remember lessons.

Other useful symptoms

Trembling hands and feet while writing.

Hungry but refuses to eat.

Averse sweet things.

< Warm food.

Nosebleed before menses.

General soreness and sensitivity. Itching, prickling, tingling all over.

Tongue paralysed.

< Company.

< Mental emotion.

CALCAREA CARBONICA

Characteristic symptoms

Nightmares.

Slow in teething and walking.

Convulsions.

Susceptible to cold.

Dull and lethargic; does not want to play.

Malnutrition.

Epilepsy.

Great weakness from excitement of walking, talking.

Ill effects of alcohol, fright.

Aversion milk, meat, fat, boiled things.

Craves eggs, sweets, dirt and indigestibles.

Ravenous hunger.

Useful mental symptoms

Overwhelmed from work and worry.

Sits and thinks about little things that amount to nothing.

Worries about responsibilities and duties.

Inability to apply himself.

Learns poorly.

Low-spirited, apathetic, apprehensive.

Depressed.

Hopeless of ever getting well.

Forgetful, confused, misplaces words, expresses himself wrongly.

Fears being observed.

Easily frightened, offended.

Cautious.
Sits and breaks sticks all day long.

Useful general symptoms

> Dry climate and weather, lying down, rubbing hands, scratching, wiping or soothing with hands, after breakfast, uncovered.

< Full moon, new moon, after midnight, at early morning, on awakening, pressure of clothes, lights, slightest change in weather.

Cannot bear sun.

CALCAREA SILICATA

Characteristic symptoms

Atrophy in children.

Epilepsy.

Aversion open air.

Sensitive to cold and draft.

Weak, emaciated and chilly.

Very sensitive generally.

Useful mental symptoms

Absent-minded.

Lacks confidence.

Fearful.

Excitable and easily angered and < anger.

Inability to concentrate on what she is reading or listening to.

Consolation irritates him.

Sits and stares into space all day and does not answer when spoken to.

Talks to people who are dead and sees dead people.

Useful general symptoms

< Change of weather, sex, cold, being overheated, motion, motion.

Aversion to food, especially meat and milk.

Great thirst.

Desires cold food and drink, milk.

Dreams of the dead, horror, frightful, murder.

Shrieking during sleep.

CANNABIS INDICA

Characteristic symptoms

Sudden loss of speech.

Fear of the dark.

Paranoia.

Inability to concentrate on one thing.

Double consciousness.

Ideas crowd upon each other.

Desires to lie down.

A great soothing remedy, in neurological disorders especially epilepsy.

Trembling.

Catalepsy.

Great anxiety, agitation and nervousness.

Epilepsy.

Extreme sensitiveness to noise. Hearing very acute. Is irritated by a whisper in next room.

Fixed gaze.

Letters run together.

Dejected expression. Weary look.

Stupid look.

Shakes head.

Shocks in brain.

Sleepy but cannot sleep. Insomnia.

Nightmares every night as soon as he falls asleep.

Bruxism in sleep. Talks in sleep. Catalepsy.

Clairvoyance and clairaudience.

Spontaneous erections.

Useful mental symptoms

Absent-minded, forgetful, cannot finish sentence.

Begins a sentence but cannot finish it.

Excessive loquacity.

Stammering and stuttering.

Exaltation of spirits.

Constant theorising.

Uncontrollable laughter.

Anguish > open air.

Paranoia.

Constant fear of insanity.

Fear of approaching death.

Useful general symptoms

Ravenous hunger, for sweets, cold drinks.

> Walking about outdoors, fresh air.

< Coffee, alcohol.

< Lying on right side, mornings.

CARCINOSINUM

Characteristic symptoms

Autism.

Allergic to foods. and chemicals. Multiple allergies.

Anticipation.

Arrested child development.

Aversion to bathing or washing.

Causations.

Chronic fatigue.

Constantly changing symptoms.

Contradictory and alternating states.

Exertion.

Grief.

Ill effects of vaccination.

Insomnia.

Loss of sleep.

Obesity.

Passionate people who over-extend themselves.

Pernicious anaemia.

Shocks, emotional.

Trembling in the morning on waking.

Vaccinations.

Windy weather.

Useful mental symptoms

Anxiety about what might happen.

Averse to reprimand or contradiction.

Deep guilty feelings.

Desire for travel.

Desires dancing and music.

Difficult concentration.

Fastidious.

Fear about crowds, exams, health.

Fear of getting cancer.

Loves thunderstorms.

Mental retardation.

OCP.

Suppression.

Sympathetic.

Other useful symptoms

Brain seems to be pulsating.

Headaches after emotion.

Food: Appetite capricious. Desires food that makes him worse.

Sleep: wakes from shocks through body. Bruxism.

Insomnia.

Never fully recovered from infection disease.

< Swimming in sea.

< Warmth of room.

> Open air, during thunderstorm.

Air of seashore agg. or amel.

Full moon agg. or amel.

New moon agg. or amel.

Approaching storm agg. or amel.

CUPRUM ACETICUM

Characteristic symptoms

Similar to Cupr. but more violent.

Brain disorders.

Chorea, periodical, with melancholy and dread of society.

Convulsions, attacks come on suddenly and periodically.

Epilepsy, with aura beginning in the knee and ascending to hypogastrium.

Facial neuralgia.

Mania.

Paralytic disorders.

Spasms.

Useful symptoms

Face, collapsed.

Facial neuralgia.

Face > chewing.

Brain seems void.

Inclined to gape, and cry.

Loses consciousness.

Head reels when in large room, vertigo in a high-ceilinged room.

Protrudes and retracts tongue. (Lach.)

Modalities

> Chewing, pressure, night, lying on affected side and warmth.

< Heat, motion, emotions, touch.

CUPRUM METALLICUM

Spasms, convulsions and cramps of violent form. Convulsions may be tonic or clonic, or during menses, during dentition, with cyanosis, from fright or emotion.

Characteristic symptoms

Hypersensitivity.

Clenches thumbs in palms.

Jerking and twitching of legs and feet.

Clonic spasms beginning in fingers and toes.

Epilepsy, aura in knees.

Paralysis of tongue, stammers, loss of speech.

Loss of speech from spasms of throat.

Deep sleep with shock beginning in limbs.

Convulsions during pregnancy and puerperal convulsions, beginning in fingers and toes and spreading.

Mental symptoms

Uneasy, morose.

Fixed ideas, malicious.

Uses words not intended.

Nervous, fearful.

Piercing shricks.

Weeps violently.

Fear of society, shuns everybody.

Confusion.

Afraid of everybody who approaches him.

Loquacious, then melancholy with fear of death.

Sense of losing consciousness.

Attacks of rage, wants to bite.

Alternating compliant and head-strong.

Imitates, mimics.

Calm obsessiveness.

Inflexibility and tension.

Tics.

Head-banging.

Useful general symptoms

Causations

Ailments from emotions, anger, fright, suppressions, overwork mentally and physically.

Ill effects of loss of sleep.

Chorea from fright.

Epilepsy from getting wet.

Modalities

> Laying hand on affected part.

> Drinking cold water.

< Emotions, fright, anger, suppressions, overwork.

< Motion.

< Loss of sleep.

< Raising arms.

< Hot weather.

< Before menses.

< At new moon.

< Touch and pressure, vomiting.

< Night.

FERRUM PHOSPHORICUM

Characteristic symptoms

Anaemia.

Emaciation.

Inflammations.

Mental lassitude.

Great physical and mental lassitude.

Indisposed to any exertion.

Nervousness.

Prostration.

Useful mental symptoms

Talkative

Hilarious, excited.

Keeps quiet.

Anger.

Transient mania from cerebral irritation.

Indifferent to pleasurable things.

Averse company.

Fear of going into a crowd.

Useful general symptoms

Jerking in limbs.

Diurnal bedwetting.

Empty feeling in head during menses.

Females: menses every three weeks.

Causalities

Ill effects of checked sweat.

Ill effects of heat and sun.

Incontinence.

Mechanical injuries.

Modalities

> Cold applications, bleeding, lying down.

< Night, 4-6 a.m.

< Touch, jar, motion.

< Right side.

< Cold air.

< Cold drinks.

< Meat, coffee, cake.

Food

Desires stimulants, sour things.

Aversion meat and milk.

Chill while eating at table.

FLUORICUM ACIDUM

Characteristic symptoms

Bone disorders, oedema.

Pale, miserable, weak types.

Chronic disease.

Compelled to move about energetically.

Always feels too hot, wants to bathe in cold water.

Discharges cause itching.

Early decay of teeth.

Late dentition.

Hair falls out.

Increased ability to exercise muscles without fatigue.

Useful mental symptoms

Must walk fast.

Needs to be on the move all the time.

Aversion to his own family.

Converses pleasantly with and is interested in strangers.

Inability to realise responsibility.

Depression.

Great lust, ogles women.

Sits silently, does not answer questions or say a word.

Useful general symptoms

Modalities

> Cold applications, cool bathing

> While walking, bending head back.

> Rapid motion.

> Eating.

< Warmth, of room, warm drinks.

< Alcohol, red wine.

< Sour foods.

< Night, morning.

GRANITE

Characteristic symptoms

Rising without cause

Has to keep moving.

Restless.

Assertiveness.

Chronic fatigue.

Pale face, strained, frowns a lot.

Sense of smell acute.

Vertigo: giddy and exhausted.

Hands trembling, trembling all over.

Sleep

Confused on waking.

Very exhausted on waking.

Unrefreshed sleep.

Dreams elderly relatives dying.

Dreams about her mother.

Aggressive dreams; she was beating people up.

Dreams of being in a war.

Violent dreams, of being raped.

Mental symptoms

Desire for company of one friend with no social interaction.

Insolent and rude.

Introversion with arrogance.

Believes that others are trivial or petty.

Outbursts of anger.

Irritability or anger at being invaded or disturbed.

Aversion to company or to socialising.

Contempt for others.

Blunt or rude and felt no care for hurting others.

Suspicious of motives of others.

Believes that others are trivial or petty.

Useful general symptoms

Limbs heavy, can hardly lift them.

Sense of smell hyperacute.

Modalities

> Lying down.

> Alcoholic drinks.

< From cold, even when hot.

< Smoking.

Food

Constant nibbling from boredom.

Can't find food she wants.

Appetite lost with nausea.

Craves sweets.

Thirsty most of the time.

HISTAMINUM

Characteristic symptoms

Quivering and cramping.

Desire to walk up and down.

Irritable and impatient.

Burning pains.

Exhaustion: does not want to move limbs at all.

Involuntary spasms and muscular contraction.

Useful mental symptoms

Insomnia with abundance of ideas.

Insomnia until 2 or 3 a.m.

Dreams of insects.

Sensitive to the slightest trifles.

Impatient, restless, with desire to move from one place to another.

Moves around aimlessly.

Quarrelsome.

Melancholy, sad.

Prostration which disappears with forced walking.

Can't stand waiting.

Pain and gastric constriction when receiving news or remembering painful experience.

Cannot find correct words, forgets proper nouns.

Slowness and difficulty understanding.

Melancholy with anguish and reduction of mental faculties.

Fears chewing in case his teeth fall out.

Useful general symptoms

Modalities

> Pressure.

> Fanning.

< Movement.

< From nervous irritation.

< From deep breathing

< Heat.

KALI BROMATUM

Characteristic symptoms

Epilepsy.

Especially when on salt free diet.

From sexual excess.

During menses.

During new moon and followed by headaches.

Nervous constitutions.

Failure of mental power.

Amnesia.

Melancholy.

Useful mental symptoms

Forgets how to talk, has to be told word before he can say it.

Amnesic aphasia.

Brain fog from grief and anxiety.

Slow, hesitates, omits or mixes up words in talking and writing.

Fidgety, busy hands, fumbles.

Moves arms about wildly.

Complains without cause.

Remorse, wrings hands, bursts into tears.

Imagines God hates him.

Paranoid delusions, of conspiracies.

Profound indifference and disgust for life.

Fears people, yet cannot remain alone in the dark.

Fear being poisoned.

Horrible illusions.

Active delirium.

Useful general symptoms

Can swallow solids easily, but not liquids.

Causations

Ill effects of worry.

Loss of business, reputation.

Embarrassment.

Illness or death of a friend.

Anger.

Fright.

Emotional disturbance.

Modalities

> Being busy physically or mentally.

< Mental exertion

< Emotions, anger.

< Fright, worry, grief.

< Periodically, at night, 2 a.m.

< Summer, new moon.

< Puberty.

< Hot weather.

< Sex, desire for.

KALI CYANATUM

Characteristic symptoms

Convulsions, epilepsy.

Tetanic convulsions with loss of consciousness.

Double vision on waking from unconsciousness.

Amnesia.

Loss of power of speech without loss of intelligence.

Useful mental symptoms

Gentle disposition.

Uncontrollably cross on entering room, though cold open air produces good mood.

Aphasia.

Inability to recollect certain words for several days.

Lying on floor in a deep stupor.

Other useful general symptoms

Modalities

> Motion in open air.

< 4 a.m. to 4 p.m.

KALI MURIATICUM

Characteristic symptoms

Habitual loss of appetite or refuses food.

Ill effects of vaccination.

Eating disorders.

Muscles of face twitch, < talking, speaking, coughing.

Stunning shock in occiput > warmth, hair let down.

Twitching in thighs.

Fatty or rich food causes indigestion.

Loss of voice, hoarseness.

Protruded appearance of eyes, with cough; feels as if eyes would come out.

Useful mental symptoms

Discontent, discouraged.

Fears evil.

Sits in silence.

Imagines he must starve.

Irritable and angry, at trifles.

Useful general symptoms

Causations

Ill effects of vaccination.

Ill effects of sprains, burns, blows, cuts.

Modalities

> Cold drinks, rubbing, letting hair down.

< Open air, cold drinks.

< Drafts, lying.

< At night.

< Dampness, sprains.

< Menses.

< Motion.

< Fatty rich food or pastry.

< Warmth of bed.

LUNA

Moon symptoms

Epilepsy < full moon. (Sil.)

Nervous afflictions, psychosis, influenced by full moon.

Moon affects ability to receive, retain, and express ideas.

< Full moon. (Alum., Calc., Graph., Nat-m. Sil. Sulph.)

Characteristic symptoms

Sleepwalking.

Oedema with neuralgia in swollen parts.

Menstrual flow amounts to haemorrhage.

Useful mental symptoms

Irritability on being spoken to.

Wants to be alone.

Mind not clear.

Disinclined to think.

Sad, depressed.

Dreams of horrible death, of murder, wakes in fright.

Useful general symptoms

Food

No appetite, slight nausea.

Desires something, she knows not what.

Immediately vomited cup of tea during headache.

Modalities

> Pains, in open air.

> Pains, cold applications.

> Belching.

LYCOPODIUM

Characteristic symptoms

Dyslexia. Spells or writes wrong words and syllables.

Cannot read what he writes.

Aphasia.

Brain fag after influenza. Incipient paralysis of brain.

Misanthropic, flies even from his children.

Suspicious.

Speech disordered.

Cramps in toes and calves at night in bed.

Twitching and jerking.

Mouth hangs open.

Diarrhoea, constipation alternate.

Sleep

On waking, becomes cross, kicks, scolds or holds his mother.

Awakes terrified.

Anxious dreams of fatal accidents.

Child sleeps all day and cries all night.

Laughs or weeps in sleep.

Useful mental symptoms

Indecision, timidity, loss of confidence.

Low self-esteem.

Fear of breaking down under stress.

Apprehensive.

Sensitive, weeps when thanked or meeting a friend.

Melancholy. Afraid to be alone.

Fear of new persons, of everything.

Anxiety as if about to die.

Headstrong and haughty when sick.

Domineering, fault finding, love for power.

Hurried when eating.

Miserly, hateful, cranky.

Failing brain power. (Anac., Bar-c., Kali-p.)

Weak memory, confused thoughts.

Useful general symptoms

Food

Aversion to bread.

Low blood sugar.

Desire sweets, pastries.

Flatulent food, cabbage, beans, onions disagree.

Likes hot food and drink.

Excessive hunger, can't stop eating.

Great weakness of digestion, belching, sour, painful.

Nodding and wagging of head.

Asthma from anger.

Causations. Ill effects of:

Fear.

Fright.

Anger.

Anxiety.

Fever.

Over-lifting.

Masturbation.

Wine.

Modalities

> By motion after midnight.
> From warm food and drink.
> On getting cold, while uncovered.
> Cold applications.
> Belching.
> Uncovering, especially head. (Sil., but Sil. must wrap up head.)
> Urinating.

< Right side from right to left, from right down.
< 4-8 p.m.
< Pressure of clothes.
< Awakening.
< Wind.
< Eating, even a little.
< Wet, stormy weather.
< Before or from suppressed menses.
< Milk, vegetables, cabbage, beans, bread, pastry.
< Heat, warm room, hot air, warm bed, warm applications, except throat and stomach (which are > warm drinks).

LYSSINUM

Characteristic symptoms

Convulsions, loss of consciousness.

Does not hear or see persons around him.

Imagines terrible things against his will.

Cannot bear heat of sun.

Thirst with inability to swallow.

Rapid speech and impatience.

Affects the nervous system.

Senses over-acute.

Convulsions from dazzling light or running water.

Irritability and dangerously violent temper.

Trembling and quivering throughout whole body.

Excitement from hearing conversation.

< Hearing water running.

Sensitivities

Hypersensitiveness of all senses.

Breath of air.

Bright objects.

Surface of water.

Sounds, especially of running water.

Thought of running water causes convulsion.

Useful mental symptoms

Fear of going mad.

Impelled to do reckless things.

Rapid speech.

Roams about.

Strange notions during pregnancy.

Rude, abusive.

Bites and strikes.

Feels he cannot endure his fears much longer.

Clairvoyance.

Useful general symptoms

Severe twitching in limbs.

Causations

Ill effects of dog bites.

Ill effects of rabies injections.

Modalities

> Bending backwards.

> Gentle rubbing.

> Steam or hot water bathing.

< Heat of sun.

< Glistening objects.

< Dazzling or reflected light.

< Wind, draft.

< Stooping.

< Bad news.

< Emotions.

< Riding in a car.

< Anything to do with running water or fluids.

MAGNESIA CARBONICA

Characteristic symptoms

Epilepsy. Myoclonic seizures: falls down suddenly while conscious.

Cannot put left foot on ground when walking.

Starts at the least sound or touch.

Spasms.

Intense neuralgia.

Nervous prostration.

Child does not thrive.

Worn out women.

Great aversion to uncovering.

Useful mental symptoms

Absent-minded, forgetful, mistakes while writing.

Anxious with perspiration all day.

Sad with indisposition to talk.

Trembling, anguish and fear as if an accident would happen, all day.

Dazed feeling.

Pack and unpacks without realising.

Insecurity and fears with trembling.

Ill-humour in evening.

> going to bed.

Useful general symptoms

Great periodicity: every second day, every third week.

Causations

Ill effects of shock, blows, mental distress, fits of passion.

Care and worry.

Pregnancy, poor feeding, milk.

Dentition, cutting wisdom teeth.

Food

Craving for meat, fruit, acids, vegetables.

Nibbles.

Aversion milk (Calc., Lyc., Sil.), vegetables, green food.

Potatoes disagree.

Violent thirst.

Modalities

> Motion, warm air, warmth of bed, waking in open air.

< Rest, especially pains: must get up and walk about.

< Change of temperature, cold, wind, weather, drafts.

< Night.

< Milk, starchy food.

NUX VOMICA

Characteristic symptoms

Brain disorders, convulsions.

Particular, zealous types.

Seems to be always out of tune.

Concentration difficult, while studying.

Confusion of mind after vexation, as if intoxicated.

Delirium in evening during nap.

Fear in the afternoon at 5 p.m.

Mistakes in measuring.

Sensitiveness to the most trifling ailments, to singing.

Hysteria.

Spasms, jerks, twists, tetanic, < slightest touch.

Sensitivities

Senses acute.

Sensitive:

- to all external impressions.
- to light.
- to music.
- before menses.
- slightest noise.
- to stepping.
- to voices.
- to rudeness.
- to sensual impressions.
- to odours.

Useful mental symptoms

Overactive mind.

Fastidious.

Fault finding, critical.

Indisposed to talk, taciturn.

Anger, when obliged to answer, when consoled.

Anxiety after eating.

Company, aversion.

Hysteria.

Imbecility.

Impatience.

Impetuous.

Indolence, aversion to work.

Irritability, consolation agg.

Maliciousness.

Mania.

Offended, easily.

Obstinate.

Quarrelsome.

Useful general symptoms

Modalities

> From a nap.

> Hot drinks, milk, fats.

< Music.

< High living.

< Sedentary habits.

< Mental exertion.

< Slight causes.

< Disappointment.

< Mental shock.

OPIUM

Characteristic symptoms

Epilepsy, convulsions.

From approach of strangers.

From glare of light.

In sleep.

From fright.

< Anger, insult, heat of room, bath.

Sleep

Sleepy but cannot sleep.

Great drowsiness.

Profound coma.

Sleeplessness from acuteness of hearing, from distant noises.

Suffocative attacks during sleep.

Twitching of limbs, one arm moves to and fro.

Insensibility of the nervous system.

Painlessness.

Lack of susceptibility to well-indicated remedies.

Useful mental symptoms

Dull, stupid, confused.

Wants nothing, says nothing is wrong.

Unable to understand or appreciate his problems.

Indifferent to pain or pleasure.

Apoplectic, unconscious, comatose.

Sees frightful visions.

Exaltations of the mind, talkative.

Tendency to lie.

Other useful general symptoms

Causations

Ill effects of fright, fear (Acon., Hyos.), anger, shame, sudden joy (Coff.), sun, rape, alcohol.

Modalities

> Cold.

> Uncovering.

> Constant walking.

< Anxiety, fear reproaches.

< Emotions, fear, fright.

< Shame.

< Joy, odours, alcohol.

< Odours.

< Alcohol.

< Suppressed discharges.

< Heat.

< During and after sleep. (Apis., Lach.)

PHOSPHORUS

Characteristic symptoms

Over-sensitive to all external impressions.

Epilepsy.

Highly nervous and sensitive.

Restless, fidgety, cannot stand still.

Great drowsiness, short naps ameliorate.

Sensation as if about to die.

Useful mental symptoms

Anxious.

Fears being alone at twilight, ghosts, the future, thunderstorms, that something is creeping towards her.

Timid and irresolute.

Amorous, uncovers body.

Excitable, impressionable.

Clairvoyant.

Weeps before menses.

Wants sympathy.

Loss of memory.

Useful general symptoms

Waterbrash.

Causations

Ill effects of anger, grief, worry, fear.

Exposure to rain, washing clothes.

Having haircut.

Modalities

> Dark.
> Cold food, cold.
> Open air.
> Sleep.
> Lying on right side.
> Washing with cold water.
> Eating.
> Massage, rubbing.
> Sitting.

< Touch.
< Warm food or drink.
< Twilight, evening.
< Change of weather, thunderstorms.
< Light.
< Emotions.
< Odours.
< Puberty.
< Physical or mental exertion, ascending stairs.
< Talking.
< Shaving.

SAMBUCUS NIGRA

Characteristic symptoms

Constant state of fretfulness.

Child wakes up suffocating and turns blue.

Dreads uncovering.

Confusion on rising.

Delirium.

Discontented with everything.

Shrieking.

Tries to escape.

Oversensitive.

Useful mental symptoms

General trembling with anxiety.

Very easily frightened.

Fright followed by suffocative attacks.

Sees images when shutting eyes.

Worse from emotions.

Useful general symptoms

Causations

Ill effects of fright, grief, anxiety.

Anxiety from fright.

Modalities

> Sitting up in bed.

> Motion.

> Wrapping up.

< Dry, cold air.

< Cold drink when overheated.

< Eating fruit.

< Sleep during rest.

< Lying down in bed.

< Motion.

< Uncovering.

SILICA

Characteristic symptoms

Epilepsy, convulsions after vaccination, aura starts in the solar plexus.

Difficult eye to eye contact.

Nervous, excitable.

Sensitive to all impressions.

Screaming violently.

Starts from slight noise.

Defective nutrition.

Ill effects of vaccination.

Pus formation.

Useful mental symptoms

Complaints from anticipation.

Loss of self-confidence. Dreads failure without reason.

Easy exhaustion.

Want of vital heat.

Yielding. Faint-hearted.

Weeping. mood.

Brain fag.

Obstinate, stubborn child.

Cries when spoken to kindly.

Obsessed with pins; searches for them and counts them.

Disgust for life, wishes to drown herself.

Cannot express herself clearly.

Fidgety.

Useful general symptoms

Causations

Loss of fluids.

Injury.

Vaccinations.

Strains.

Foreign objects.

Overwork, mental or physical.

Modalities

> Warm room, wraps, warmth, summer.

> Profuse urination.

< Change of weather, cold, air, drafts, damp.

< Uncovering, bathing.

< Mental exertion, talking.

< Nervous excitement.

> Light, noise, touch, pressure.

< Combing hair.

< Washing during menses.

< Lying down.

< Early morning.

< New moon and full moon.

STAPHYSAGRIA

Characteristic symptoms

Nervous disorders with trembling.

Ill effects of anger, humiliation, guilt and shame.

Marked irritability.

Morbidly sensitive.

Ill effects of scolding and punishment in children.

Very sensitive about what others will say about him.

Useful mental symptoms

Violent outbursts of passion.

Always angry, gloomy, petulant.

Throws things.

Peevish. Child cries for many things but refuses them.

Poor memory.

Prefers solitude.

Sensitive in every way.

Hypochondriacal, sad.

Imagines insults.

Great indignation about what others have done to him

Useful general symptoms

Causations

Ill effects of anger and insults.

Anger suppressed or reserved.

Humiliation.

Mercury.

Dentition.

Rape, surgery, sexual abuse.

Modalities

> After breakfast.

> Warmth.

> From rest at night.

> Sex.

< Anger, indignation, grief.

< Sexual excess.

< Least touch.

< Night, new moon, before full moon.

STRAMONIUM

Characteristic symptoms

Chorea, epilepsy, from fright.

Convulsions < night.

Hysteria.

Weeping.

Catalepsy.

Tonic and clonic spasms, alternately.

Delusions as to size and distance.

Rhythmic movements of head and arms.

Spasms from shiny things and water. (Lyss.)

Useful mental symptoms

Hallucinations.

Fixed ideas.

Must have light and company; can't bear solitude or darkness.

Ceaseless talking.

Raving mania.

Useful general symptoms

Causations

Ill effects of shock, fright, sun, childbirth, fever.

Modalities

> Bright light.

> Company.

> Warmth.

> Mirror.

> Surface of water.

< Cloudy days.

< Touch.

< Fright.

< Suppressions.

< Dark room.

< When alone after sleep.

< On swallowing.

< Pressure.

< Sun.

< Shiny objects, water.

SULPHUR

Characteristic symptoms

Epilepsy.

Mania.

Aversion to meat.

Desires sweets.

Milk disagrees.

Drinks much, eats little.

Children old-looking.

Great irritability.

Useful mental symptoms

Irritable.

Depressed.

Egotistical.

Obstinate.

Intellectual.

Busy all the time.

Absent-minded, misplaces words.

Selfish.

Useful general symptoms

Causations

Suppressions.

Alcohol.

Sun.

Over-exertion.

Modalities

> Dry, warm weather, dry heat.

> Open air, motion.

> Seating, walking.

< At rest.

< Warmth of bed.

< Washing and bathing in morning.

< 11 a.m.

< Night.

< Suppressions.

< Milk.

TARENTULA HISPANICA

Characteristic symptoms

Depression, insanity, mania, sexual mania.

Chorea.

Highly strung.

Nervous phenomena.

Extreme restlessness.

Violence.

Excitement from music.

Destructive impulses.

Lacks control.

Erratic.

Impulsive.

Feigns fainting, insensibility.

In constant motion even though walking agg.

Restless, fidgety, hurried.

Rolls on ground from side to side.

Quivering, jerking, trembling, twitching.

Irregular movements.

Useful mental symptoms

Sudden alteration of moods.

Fits of nervous laughter, then screaming.

Lacks control, erratic, impulsive.

Destructive, tears her clothes.

Throws things away.

Calmer when there are no observers.

Angry with despair.

Melancholy, discontented.

Useful general symptoms

Causations

Ill effects of bad news.

Scolding.

Punishment.

Modalities

> Open air.

> Music.

> Bright colours.

> Pressure, rubbing affected parts.

> Motion.

> Warm water.

> Relaxation.

< Rest.

< Periodically, at the same hour.

< Touch.

< Cold, damp.

< Night, evening.

< After menses.

< Sex.

< Motion, contact, noises seeing others in trouble.

< Washing hands in cold water.

THUJA

Characteristic symptoms

Complaints after vaccination, never well since.

Speech slow, hunts for words.

Over excited, angry.

Rapid exhaustion and emaciation.

Fixed ideas.

Dullness of mind.

Catalepsy

Epilepsy.

Asthma in children.

Sweats only on uncovered parts.

Useful mental symptoms

Dreams of death, of falling from a height.

Insomnia.

Hurried with ill humour.

Talks hastily, swallows words.

Fixed ideas, as if a stranger were at his side.

Emotional sensitiveness, music causes weeping and trembling.

Sadness. Aversion to life.

Dullness of mind, cannot concentrate.

Speech slow, hunts for words.

Quarrelsome to family, but not to others.

Over-excited, angry, anxious about trifles.

Post-natal depression.

Walks in circle in room.

Useful general symptoms

Twitching, weakness and trembling.

Limbs feel as if they would break easily.

Feels cold, dread, on waking at night.

Knees restless.

Causations

Suppressed gonorrhoea.

Vaccinations.

Sunstroke.

Tea, coffee, beer, sweets, fat, onions.

Mercury.

Modalities

> Drawing up limbs.

> Warmth, air, wind.

> Sneezing.

> Motion.

> Crossing legs.

> Pressure, rubbing, scratching.

< Periodically.

< Increasing moonlight.

< Menses.

< Urinating, chewing, stretching, sex, closing eyes.

< Touch.

< After breakfast, eating.

< Sun, bright light.

Food

Complete loss of appetite.

Aversion fresh meat, potatoes, onions and garlic.

Cannot eat onions.

Dyspepsia from drinking tea.

Unable to eat breakfast.

Desires cold drinks.

Desires salt.

TUBERCULINUM

Characteristic symptoms

Epilepsy.

Lowe recuperative powers.

Susceptible to changes in weather.

Mentally deficient children.

Catches cold easily, on slightest exposure.

Useful mental symptoms

Desire to travel, does not want to stay in one place for long.

Wants to do something different, find a new doctor.

Weary of life.

Reckless.

Depressed, melancholy, hopeless.

Anxious, whines and complains about little things.

Contradictory behaviour, changing moods.

Fits of violent temper, wants to fight, throws things at anyone.

Sensitive to music.

Aversion to mental work.

Confused, everything in the room seems strange.

Child has nightmares.

Useful general symptoms

Loquacious during fever.

Modalities

> Open air, cool wind.

< Noise music, standing.

< Change of weather.

< Periodically.

< On waking.

< Evening, after dinner.

VERATRUM ALBUM

Characteristic symptoms

Profound mentals.

Violent mania alternates with silence and refusal to talk.

Faints from least emotion, exertion.

Convulsions from excitement, of children.

Useful mental symptoms

Melancholy, head hangs down, broods in silence, wants to be alone.

Melancholy with stupor and mania.

Sits stupidly, notices nothing.

Sullen indifference.

Aimlessly wandering around house.

Manic desire to tear things. (Tarent.)

Sings, whistles, laughs.

Tells others of their faults.

Imaginary disease.

Useful general symptoms

Causations

Post-operative shock, shock of injury.

Ill effects of fright, disappointed love, injured pride.

Suppressed rashes.

Alcohol.

Modalities

> Children being carried quickly.

> Walking around.

> Hot drinks.

< Night.

< Before and during menses, stools.

< Worse touch, pressure.

< Injured pride.

ZINCUM METALLICUM

Characteristic symptoms

Nervous constitution.

Automatic motions of the hands, arms, mouth.

Convulsive twitching, jerking, spasms.

Great relief from discharges.

Convulsions with pale face and no heat.

Chorea from fright.

Fidgety feet, trembling, twitching.

Useful mental symptoms

Muddled.

Brain fag.

Weak memory.

Very sensitive noise.

Averse work, talk.

Fretful, peevish, cries if vexed or moved during sleep (children).

Child repeats everything said to it.

Melancholia.

Lethargic, stupid.

Easily startled or excited.

Forgetful.

Screams with pain.

Sensitive to others talking and to noise.

Stares on waking as if frightened, rolls head from side to side.

Weeps when angry.

Thinks of death calmly.

Useful general symptoms

Causations

Chorea from fright, worse sleep.

Ill effects of fright, grief, anger.

Ill effects of surgery.

Ill effects of study.

Ill effects of concussion.

Ill effects of suppressions.

Ill effects of otorrhoea.

Ill effects of menses.

Modalities

> Eating.

> Appearance of eruptions.

> Motion, hard pressure, rubbing, scratching.

> Warm open air.

> Free discharges, menses.

< Being touched.

< Noise.

< Sweet things.

< Being touched during menstrual period.

Appendix 1 Gut Dysbiosis

Gastrointestinal problems are experienced by almost all autistics, especially children, and there is a direct correlation between the severity of an autistic presentation and the severity of gastrointestinal issues. Such concomitants as headache, noise sensitivity, and irritability, are all usually related to constipation, diarrhoea and abdominal pain.[13]

Manifestations of Gut Dysbiosis

The manifestations of leaky gut syndrome may include:

arthritis - joint pain
autoimmune disease
brain issues, e.g., brain fog
chronic fatigue syndrome

---

[13] An excellent reference on the subject is Campbell-McBride, Natasha, *Gut and Psychology Syndrome*, Medinform Publishing, Soham, Cambridge, 2004.

cravings, especially for carbohydrates
digestive problems
immune system disorders
multiple allergies
neurological disorders
nutritional deficiencies
skin rashes.

Leaky gut syndrome must be addressed at the very beginning of homoeopathic treatment. If dietary steps are to be taken, they must run alongside homoeotherapy. They will change the total symptom picture. However, they will make clearer what may be achieved.

The steps that must be taken are quite simple, and advice is within the purview of the homoeopath.

Leaky gut as pseudochronic disease

We always think of gut dysbiosis as the result of a pseudochronic disease, in other words, one that has a maintaining cause. Therefore, in addition to addressing homoeopathically the patient's anxiety, we have to give some consideration to the improving the bowel flora. I have found that the prescription of Candida Albicans in potency often and for a lengthy period, together with a hepatoprotective remedy, for example, Lycopodium, in a widely different potency. If it is known that there is a specific other overgrowth of bowel flora, consideration should be given to prescribing that in potency as well.

Dietary Measures

Certain non-homoeopathic steps might be considered.

Remove: low-to-no-value foods

breakfast foods

butter substitutes

delicatessen meats

grains and related products

lactose-containing products

processed foods

snack foods

soya

starchy beans and peas

starchy food

sugar

Add high-value foods

all fresh and frozen meats

fat on meat

filtered water and mineral water

for adults: tea (including herbal tea) and coffee

fruit, especially avocados

mushrooms

non-starchy beans and pulses

non-starchy vegetables

virgin cold-pressed oils

Vegetarianism

Many autistic children are anaemic, and should not be placed on a vegetarian diet, as it might impair bone and muscle development and neurological development.

Dietary supplements

a high quality probiotic
digestive enzymes
essential fatty acids
vitamin A
vitamin and mineral supplements as judged advisable, especially Magnesium and Zinc.

Appendix 2 Some Famous Autistics

A few well-known autistic figures in history and currently.

Alan Turing
Albert Einstein
Andy Warhol
Anthony Hopkins
Beethoven
Bill Gates
Bobby Fischer
Charles Darwin
Courtney Love
Dan Aykroyd
Daryl Hannah
Elon Musk
Emily Dickinson
Friedrich Nietzsche
George Orwell
H.G. Wells
Hans Christian Andersen
Henry Cavendish
Henry Ford
James Joyce

Jane Austen
Jerry Seinfeld
Julian Assange
Lewis Carroll
Ludwig Wittgenstein
Mark Twain
Michael Jackson
Michelangelo
Nikola Tesla
Paul Dirac
Satoshi Tajiri
Sir Alfred Hitchcock
Sir Isaac Newton
Stanley Kubrick
Steve Jobs
Temple Grandin
Thomas Edison
Thomas Jefferson
Tim Burton
Vincent Van Gogh
William Butler Yeats
Mozart

Glossary

A

Actual medical power The product of a remedy's intrinsic curative power and its nominal numerical potency.

Aggravation 1. **Allopathic a.** Iatrogenic poisoning. 2. **Homoeopathic a.** An acute transient episode of the presenting symptoms following homoeopathic medication. It is due to an apparent acceleration of the life force in the direction of the desuppression. **3. Isopathic a.** An aggravation of symptoms following the administration of an isopathic medicine. It is due to a proving of the **vector**. 4. **Constitutional a.** Transient symptomatic amplification following administration of the **constitutional**.

Amplificational mode Mode of medicinal action in which the patient exhibits an increase in vitality (resulting in aggravation, if symptomatology exists), often seen after the constitutional is administered.

Antidote A remedy that has been selected for the purpose of neutralising the ill-effects of a remedy which has been incorrectly prescribed.

Ascending collective dose A form of **collective dose** in which the potency is fractionally increased before each administration.

B

Burnout Complete exhaustion as the result of overwhelm, usually due to the effort of passing, with inability to make decisions.

C

Chronic disease A cycle of similar acute illnesses with a constant background of pain, dysfunction or immobility at any or all levels of eccentricity.

Chronicity 1. The time elapsed since the onset of symptoms. **2. C of symptoms**. A result of the failure of the life force to complete its timely expression through the organism.

Collective dose A dose of a given potentialised medicine, when dispensed as a set of exposures.

Concurrent medication The prescribing of two or more remedies without waiting for the action of each remedy to be exhausted.

Concurrent remedies Remedies whose courses of action at least partly coincide.

Constitution The complete organism in all of its spheres: behavioural, intellectual, emotional, physical, being the sum of all that it has inherited and acquired.

Constitutional diathesis The features of a given constitution that leads it to be susceptible to specific morbific agents or influences and predisposed to specific forms of illness.

Constitutional prescribing Prescribing a remedy that matches the patient's apparent constitutional picture, for the purpose of amplifying the patient's vital force.

Constitutional, -al remedy A remedy that is reminiscent of the constitution of a patient.

Curative action The action of a medicine as the result of its resemblance to the presenting symptoms.

Curative mode A mode of medicinal action in which the similimum acts.

Cure The complete removal of an illness state, including the removal of the primary disturbance-resistance complex.

D

Deconcentration **1.** A **potency** whose creation has involved placing a small quantity of a **mother tincture** (or **mother power**) into a larger quantity of a ritually used substance, usually water. **2.** This process (classical: *dilution*).

Degree of chronicity The time elapsed since the highest degree of symptoms first appeared.

Detoxification Drainage. The elimination from the organism of toxins that have become obstacles to cure, using potentised remedies, especially isopathically. It includes the elimination of any toxins that it is within the power of the medicine to remove, where a toxin is defined as anything physical or non-physical that naturally causes the vital force to become distorted or stalled.

Detoxification combination A combination of (usually two) medicines used in a detoxification strategy, consisting of: an ***initiator or elimination remedy*** (the remedy prescribed in the higher potency) and a ***support (or protective remedy*** (the remedy prescribed in the lower potency). These **concurrent**

remedies are prescribed as two separate simplexes, giving control over the adjustment of dosage.

Detoxification strategy A plan for detoxifying a patient, typically involving the prescription of a **detoxification combination** together with appropriate supporting measures, e.g., lifestyle adjustment.

Disturbance Disturbance of the life force. Resistance. It is disturbance of the life force that causes the organism to become diseased.

Divided dose dispensing The extempore dispensing, often by a carer, of a **collective dose** at an experimental low potency, to induce initial susceptibility while controlling aggravation. Typically, this kind of dosing would be performed often, and by sipping from a glass, with succussion by stirring.

Dosage The amount of exposure to a medicine.

Dose A single exposure or collection of exposures to a given potentialised medicine.

E

Elimination response An increase in the elimination of toxins, often accompanied by symptoms.

Eliminative mode Mode of medicinal action in which the patient exhibits increased mental and emotional activity, with physiological elimination. The primary mode of **isopathy**.

Epidemic prescribing Prescribing with a view to eliminating a group disease. It is facilitated by the association of certain remedies with group syndromes (especially in the case of the infectious diseases) that are all manifestations of group syndromes and have their own associated remedies.

Euthenic, euthenic therapy In **obstetric homoeopathy**, the use of an isopathics to remove the influence of a group disease from the mother.

Extended divided dose dispensing **Divided dose dispensing** with the additional dimension of deconcentration, done by placing a drop of the medicine in a fresh glass of water, before stirring and dispensing.

F

Family of remedies A group of remedies having a common set of distinctive symptoms.

G

Group disease A disease of a group. It corresponds, by a factor of scale, to an individual disease. *See* **miasm theory**.

Group disease remedy A signature remedy which is evoked by the diseased group from nature (the externality to which it aspires), and which belongs to the family of isopathics.

Group disease vector A communicable noxious influence whose establishment in the individual signals acceptance of disease.

Group syndrome The symptomatology of a **group disease**.

H

Healing gradient **1.** The natural inclination of the organism to heal. **2.** The inclination to heal that is installed when a potentialised medicine is administered.

Healing characteristics theorem Radiant healing occurs with the characteristics of the life force.

I

Incurable illness **1.** In homoeopathic medicine, disease in which the dominant aetiology-symptomatology complex cannot be resolved, usually because of an obstacle to the curative routine. **2.** Disease in which there has been virtual destruction of a vital organ.

Indirect elimination The elimination of toxins which is routinely achieved as a by-product of homoeotherapy.

Initiator remedy In a detoxification combination, the remedy prescribed in the higher potency, usually an isopathic designed to initiate and maintain elimination of a group disease vector.

Intercurrent remedy A remedy prescribed for an apparently unrelated acute symptom picture that appears during treatment of a chronic disease.

Isopathic Of a medicine, being made from the same species that caused the disease.

Isopathic prescribing The prescribing of a homoeopathic medicine on the principle that a specific and not generic (that is, similar) match will result in the annihilation of a form of resistance that is identifiable with a group disease. Isopathics are often prescribed for the elimination of group disease **morphogenetic fields**, and with them, group disease vectors, leading to partial or specific detoxification of the individual.

Isopathy Treatment of group disease by administering a potentised group disease vector.

M

Maintaining cause The sustaining factor in a case of **pseudo-chronic disease**.

Masking Changing one's personality to conform to social pressure.

Materia medica **1.** The contents of the homoeopathic pharmacy. **2.** ***Homoeopathic Materia Medica*** The published summaries of provings and related information.

Meltdown Uncontrollable loss of emotional equanimity on the scale of a tantrum.

Miasmic A remedy that is strongly associated with a specific miasm, e.g., Nitricum Acidum; Syphilinum (luetic miasm).

Modality **1.** An ameliorating or aggravating factor. **2.** A therapeutic approach. **3.** A remedial display of modal dynamics, e.g., cure.

Modes of medicinal response There are eight: amplificational, curative, eliminative, palliative, probative, restorative, supportive, and susceptive. (See each, separately.)

Morphic field Resonant field. See **morphogenetic field**.

Morphic resonance Harmonic attunement resulting in reverberative propagation, and synchronisation.

Morphogenetic field A self-organising and self-remembering, spatio-temporal, vibratory, pattern-imposing, probabilistic field shared by co-resonating members.

N

Neurotypical A neurologically normal human.

Nosode A remedy prepared from a pathological product.

O

Order of cure In the holistic medical strategy, the order is: first, the removal of obstacles to cure; second, detoxification; third, homoeotherapy as indicated by the symptomatology most in evidence or emphasised, including aetiology.

Order of healing theorem As healing progresses pathology retrogresses.

P

Palliation The use of homoeopathic medicines to relieve suffering, without the expectation of cure.

Palliative mode A mode of medicinal action designed to bring about rapid relief.

Passing Presenting oneself as neurotypical.

Plain face A deadpan expression commonly seen in autistics when not masking.

Plussing The practice of succussing a medicine before it is dispensed, usually by succussing the medicine bottle 5-10 times, for the purpose of increasing its potency.

Posoequivalence theorem A single disturbance of the life force will call for a single dose of the medicine that will initiate cure.

Posology The study of dosage. In homoeopathy it is concerned solely with the measure of the patient's exposure to the remedy.

Potency Curative power.

Potency selection The creation of a potency that will match the patient's resistance to the flow of the vital force, thereby annihilating it.

Potentialisation A process by which the essential healing nature of a remedy is transformed into a curative power or esoteric medicine.

Potentisation The initial pharmaceutical process of serial deconcentration and succussion of a sacrificially prepared essence, usually for the purpose of carrying out an experimental proving or preparing off-shelf-potencies.

Probative mode Mode of medicinal action in which a proving of the remedy occurs.

Prophylaxis Homoeopathic prescribing in anticipation of a disturbance of the vital force.

Proving **1.** The experimental process of discovering an essence's intrinsic curative powers by medication with the essence in potency. **2.** Unintended or accidental manifestation of a remedy's symptom picture following clinical medication.

Pseudo-chronic disease A category of disease that resembles chronic disease but always is sustained by repeated exposures to a morbific agent.

R

Remedy A potential solution to a medical problem.

Repertory The separately published index to the ***Homoeopathic Materia Medica***.

Restorative mode Mode of medicinal action following homoeotherapy in which the patient's post-curative life changes for the better.

S

Shutdown A complete loss of activity, resembling depressive episode.

Special interest Something an autistic takes an interest in to the point of obsession.

Species analogue Similimum. An essence that resembles a given disturbance-resistance complex in its symptomatogenicity.

Split dose A dose of a homoeopathic medicine that anticipates an interruption, e.g., sleep. It is given before and after the interruption.

Stimming Self-stimulating behaviour, typically leg movements or hand movements used to reduce stress.

Succussion A stage of **potentisation**, consisting of imparting serial shocks to a solution to 'potentise' or 'dynamise' it. The effect is to set the phase of the potency.

Support remedy In a detoxification combination, the remedy prescribed in the lower potency, usually for the support and protection of organs of elimination.

Susceptibility The ability to be infected by a given group influence or vector, including a known remedy. Clinically, susceptibility may be instilled, enhanced or made permanent.

Susceptive mode Mode of medicinal action in which remedy acceptability, both immediate and persisting, is enhanced or instilled.

Symptom A datum elicited from the patient concerning illness. Symptoms include: complaints; clinical signs; the results of laboratory pathology tests; observations, including the observations of witnesses.

T

Totality of the case The totality of the case comprises the patient's presenting problem and its symptoms, what is to be cured, and the dimensions of the disturbance of the patient's vital energy.

Treatment strategy A plan for individual treatment, counselling, review, treatment support and patient advice.

V

Vaccinosis The generic group disease caused by **vaccination**.

Vital force The life force. That which expresses itself in the world.

Vortexing Ritual stirring done for the purpose of raising the increasing the phase of a potency.

About the Author

Peter Twohig BA, BA (Hons), BHlthSc (Hom), DHeal, ND (Adv), DHom *NC*, DHom *AIH*, GrDHomMed, MAIH

Peter is formerly a director of Littlewood Clinic of Homoeopathic and Energistic Medicine in Crows Nest, Sydney, and a lecturer at several colleges in Sydney.

Prior to practising medicine, Peter had a career in management consulting and computer system development. Peter's career in healing began when he became a Reiki channel. He eventually met channels who also worked in other fields, and was introduced to homoeopathy, naturopathy, neurolinguistic programming (NLP), past life therapy, and psychic healing. He has since given up his medical practice in order to concentrate on writing.

Peter is also an award-winning fiction writer and poet. He comes from Melbourne, but now lives in sunny Central Coast, New South Wales, and is interested in, well, everything.

Drop into my website:

WildHomoeopathy.com, where you'll find a blog, and lots of further reading and news of projected works.

Books by Peter Twohig

LITERARY FICTION

The Richmond Trilogy

The Cartographer

The Torch

The Mazemaster

Other novels

An Ill-fitting Man (Out in 2023)

SCIENCE FICTION

The Messiah Trilogy

The Last Messiah (Out in 2023)

BOOKS FOR HOMOEOPATHS

A Vitalistic Approach to Homoeopathic Medicine

Case Management as a Clinical Technology

Introduction to Isopathic Prescribing

The Homoeopathic Approach to Autism

Welcome to Homoeopathy! (Out in 2022)

THE HOMOEOPATHY 2.0 SERIES (Out Now)[14]

Homoeopathy is undergoing a rebirth. At the same time, a world-wide explosion of interest in alternative medicine and healing technologies is taking place. In the spirit of this movement, the Homoeopathy 2.0 series of books has arrived.

The complete Homoeopathy 2.0 series of three books will:

- provide you with a deeper understanding of the philosophy of homoeopathy, thereby diminishing its mystique
- reveal a multitude of ways to use potentialised medicines, both singly and in combination to achieve results
- offer modern and common-sense formulations of homoeopathic concepts that can be used to adopt sound and logical prescribing habits
- show you how to bring to bear a battery of prescribing techniques and theories to help you create a more confident clinical practice
- recontextualise your training and experience within a vitalistic framework, thus enabling you to reconnect with a workable classical view

---

[14] The Homoeopathy 2.0 series of books is published by Warburton Press, Wyoming NSW, and is available on Amazon.

- explain why potencies behave the way they do, and how to use that knowledge in the clinic.
- clarify vague concepts of, for example, potency election, constitutional remedies, detoxification, miasms, antidoting, aggravation, and prophylaxis supply you with the means to deal with the issues of modern homoeopathy once and for all.

Book 1 - A Vitalistic Approach to Homoeopathic Medicine

This book provides:

- an outline of the principles of vitalistic medicine as they relate to homoeopathy
- a revised homoeopathic pharmacodynamic system
- a revision, along classical lines, of homoeopathic theory, and an outline of its clinical applications.

Book 2 - Case Management as a Clinical Technology

This book provides:

- an implementation of the principles enunciated in Book 1 specially designed to achieve improved results in cases of chronic disease
- case analysis, repertorising, and potency and dosage selection advice from the first consultation to the final review
- strategies and therapeutic guidelines for the management of notoriously difficult cases types.

Book 3 - Introduction to Isopathic Prescribing

This book provides:

- a theory of group disease (including its displacement of miasmic theory)
- an introduction to the principles of isopathic technology using potentised remedies
- strategies and therapeutic guidelines for the management of detoxification
- strategies and therapeutic guidelines for the management of prophylaxis
- a set of palliative protocols for treating certain categories of commonly seen disorders.

Acknowledgements

Thanks go to my fabulous sister Kate for her suggestions and help in preparing the cover design for publication.

Many thanks to Elizabeth Sanford for reading the text.

Made in United States
Orlando, FL
04 November 2026

90201377R00154